Long After I'm Gone

Based on conversations between a man and his daughter in the final months of his life: by Deborah Good with sections by Nelson Good, as told to and interpreted by Deborah.

Long After I'm Gone

A Father-Daughter Memoir

Deborah Good
with Nelson Good

Foreword by
John Stahl-Wert

DreamSeeker Books
TELFORD, PENNSYLVANIA

an imprint of
Cascadia Publishing House

Copublished with
Herald Press
Scottdale, Pennsylvania

Cascadia Publishing House orders, information, reprint permissions:
contact@CascadiaPublishingHouse.com
1-215-723-9125
126 Klingerman Road, Telford PA 18969
www.CascadiaPublishingHouse.com

Long After I'm Gone

DreamSeeker Books is an imprint of Cascadia Publishing House
Copublished with Herald Press, Scottdale, PA
Library of Congress Catalog Number: 2008048685
ISBN 13: 978-1-931038-55-3; **ISBN 10:** 1-931038-55-4
Book design by Cascadia Publishing House
Cover design by Dawn Ranck; Nelson and Deborah Good atop Mount
Washington in New Hampshire, 1991. Photo credit: Betty Good.

🔁 ∞™

The paper used in this publication is recycled and meets the
minimum requirements of American National Standard for Information Sciences—
Permanence of Paper for Printed Library Materials, ANSI Z39.48-1984.1984

All Bible quotations are used by permission, all rights reserved and unless otherwise noted are from *The New Revised Standard Version of the Bible*, copyright
1989, by the Division of Christian Education of the National Council of the
Churches of Christ in the USA

Library of Congress Cataloguing-in-Publication Data
Good, Deborah.
  Long after I'm gone : a father-daughter memoir / Deborah Good with Nelson
Good ; foreword by John Stahl-Wert.
    p. cm.
  Summary: "Here a father's history-telling combines with a daughter's personal
journey of remembrance, loss, and grief. The voice of Nelson Good intertwines
with that of his young adult daughter, Deborah Good, as he fights the cancer
that will kill him while telling her the stories of seven projects, communities,
and organizations he had cared about"--Provided by publisher.
  ISBN-13: 978-1-931038-55-3 (5.5 x 8.5 trade pbk. : alk. paper)
  ISBN-10: 1-931038-55-4 (5.5 x 8.5 trade pbk. : alk. paper)
  1. Mennonites--United States--Biography. 2. Fathers and daughters--United
States. 3. Cancer--Patients--Washington (D.C.)--Biography. 4. Washington
(D.C.)--Biography. 5. Washington (D.C.)--Church history. 6. Mennonite
Church--History--20th century. 7. Community life--Washington (D.C.) 8.
Oral history--United States. I. Good, Nelson, d. 2005. II. Good, Deborah. III.
Title.
  E184.M45G64 2009
  306.874'2--dc22
                                    2008048685

16 15 14 13 12 11 10 09   10 9 8 7 6 5 4 3 2 1

In memory of Nelson W. Good
May 16, 1944 – July 13, 2005

CONTENTS

FOREWORD

Long After I'm Gone is, at its heart, a love story. The life-tested wisdom of the late Nelson Good interweaves with the soul-rich reflections of his poet-daughter Deborah to produce a deeply resonant chronicle of a father, of a father and his daughter, and of the ever-widening circles of loving influence that ripple out from this truly special man.

It must be pointed out that, were Nelson still alive, he would already be protesting. The too-easy attribution of "wisdom" to himself, he would patiently explain, wry grin and smiling eyes on full display, is the common mistake of the historian who wants to retrospectively assign brilliance where it would not have fit the stumble-along life as it was actually lived. His modesty in this regard would not be false; "Good" might have been his name, but Nelson knew that goodness came *to* him— maybe *through* him—but not *from* him.

Nelson Good was the truest "servant leader" I have ever known. His mentor, Robert Greenleaf, famously asked this question of servant leaders: "Do those served grow as persons; do they, while being served, become healthier, wiser, freer, more autonomous, more likely themselves to become servants?" Deborah's chronicle of her dad's life provides stories of just this result. Those touched by Nelson rose up to wholeness, wisdom, freedom, capability, and the kind of beauty Nelson himself exhibited, the beauty of powerful, selfless effectuality.

But beyond her chronicle, it is Deborah—Deborah the writer of this beautiful book, Deborah the daughter of this beautiful man—who shows us her father best. Her courage, vulnerability, eloquence, and grace shine as she shares her pride and her grief in her father's life and death.

Nelson Good was a builder of prototypes—of models— and he continuously reworked his practical experiments for human living. He discerned, thirty years ahead of the curve, that it wasn't society that was breaking down so much as it was community that had been abandoned. Discerning this, he set upon the task of shaping community spaces in which humans could grow as persons and forge purposeful relationships. He did this work quietly, steadily, against the odds, fruitful decade after fruitful decade. The full extent of Nelson's "loving influence" will never be known, as its impact is ongoing.

In my own case, if you pull on the thread that was the contribution Nelson Good made to the weaving of my life, everything I currently understand and do comes undone. This isn't whimsy. It would be a denial of life's grace for me to say otherwise. It would be un-Nelson-like.

Long After I'm Gone is, most deeply, a love story about the servanthood of God—the humility of God, if you will—in raising us up into our own personhood, into loving community, and into common cause with our companions. Nelson Good, modest as he was on this subject especially, gave us one of our very best glimpses yet of this deeper story. Deborah Good's love for this man, as captured in her interviews with her father and in her narratives, has now become a grace to all of us through the gift of this book.

—*John Stahl-Wert, Pittsburgh, Pennsylvania, is father of two daughters, president of Pittsburgh Leadership Foundation, 1977-1978 alumnus of Nelson Good's WSSY Program, and internationally best-selling author of four books, including* The Serving Leader.

PROLOGUE:
A NOTE FROM THE
DAUGHTER

In 2004, Dad sent me a card for my twenty-fourth birthday. *Thank you for being there for me,* it read, *and for us as parents. . . . I'm looking forward to being with you this weekend. Might you stay awhile?*

At the time, I could have found it funny that he would thank me for "being there" for him when usually he was taking care of me, not the other way around. We had no way of knowing that our roles would change significantly just a few months later, and that by the time my twenty-fifth birthday came around, he would be gone.

My dad, Nelson Weaver Good, born and raised on a farm in Mennonite Lancaster County, Pennsylvania, had lived in Washington, D.C., for more than thirty-five years when he was diagnosed with adrenocortical cancer at the end of January 2005. His back had been hurting for about two weeks—his first real symptom. After many doctor's visits and several diagnoses, we learned the horrifying reason for his pain.

I was standing beside Dad's stretcher at Washington Hospital Center when his assigned doctor approached us with the news. The CT-scan taken two hours earlier, she said, showed a large mass on his left adrenal gland and spots in his lungs and liver. It was, we would learn, a rare and aggressive cancer that had silently spread from his left adrenal gland to his lungs, liver, and bones.

In the tumultuous week that followed, I quit a part-time job I had in Philadelphia and decided to stay in Washington indefinitely.

The news threw our family into a terrible, beautiful, and unpredictable storm that tossed us about, ripped at our hearts, and pushed our relationships to new depths. We spent hours together, laughed and cried, and told each other, "I love you" more than we ever had before.

Over the next five and a half months, Ryan, my older brother, and his wife, Hannah, traveled many miles back and forth between their home in Indiana and Washington, D.C. They had been married less than one month when Dad was diagnosed. My younger brother, Jason, made frequent trips to D.C. while finishing his senior year at nearby Eastern Mennonite University, sometimes bringing his girlfriend Bryn with him, and then moved home for the last two months of Dad's life.

Meanwhile, my mom, Betty, and I cared for Dad as best we knew. Dad stretched out in the front seat on the way to his many medical appointments. He underwent radiation and chemotherapy, but by May, it was clear treatments were not working. Two months later, the cancer had carved bowls in his cheeks and temples; his arms were emaciated, his legs swollen with fluid. And on July 13, his miserable body finally let him go. He was sixty-one years old.

In late April, we had no prognosis but were very aware of the disease's heavy hand and its threat to Dad's life. The daily reminders of his mortality—and my own—nudged me into reflection, thinking about the depth of perspective and story he carried inside him. Was there any way I could hold on to just a little of that wisdom in a more permanent way?

I realized one thing I wished for: I wanted to hear Dad tell his story of developing the Washington Study-Service Year (WSSY) program. The program was his brainchild back in 1976 and still exists today, bringing students from Mennonite colleges to live, work, and study together in D.C. I remember WSSY students babysitting me as a child, and, much later, I myself participated in the program as a college senior in 2002.

I suggested that I interview Dad about the program's beginnings and record it on audiocassette. He was open to the idea, and as we talked together about it, this seed grew into a much larger proposal. Dad thought he might enjoy an opportunity to reflect not only on the WSSY program but on other pieces of his adult life.

We decided that Dad and I would have conversations about seven different projects and communities with which he had been involved: Friendship Flat, WSSY, the FLOC Learning Center, Rolling Ridge, Community House Church, the Thurgood Marshall Center, and then WSSY once again, this time with a new name: the Washington Community Scholars' Center (WCSC). We would record the interviews onto audiocassettes, and I would then transcribe and edit the interviews so they could be read by others.

The project would give Dad something purposeful to do when unable to do much else. Mom and others would also value having some of this history preserved, and I had the time, energy, and writing experience to make it happen. I was thrilled.

Over the next two months, Dad and I sat together seven different times with a tape recorder between us. He rested in a simple green recliner, on loan from a friend, which we had lined with foam padding to reduce his pain. He propped his head on pillows and moistened his mouth with water from a bottle at his side. Every so often, a timer would go off in the kitchen, and I'd hop up from where I sat with a notebook on my lap to get his medications.

I usually let Dad begin the conversation. As he talked, I asked questions to clarify or to reach for more detail. Often, we broke away from the chronological story to delve into analysis of this or that: Sometimes he described in more detail organizational and community models, or we discussed the values that formed a foundation beneath his work. This analysis was the part I loved.

From a young age, I remember riding back with Dad from soccer games or church retreats and reflecting out loud about social dynamics—how groups of people related to each other, how girl athletes were treated differently from boys, how kids at school divided themselves along race lines.

Through these conversations, Dad taught me to not only participate in the world but to observe and analyze it. When I went to college in 1998, I, like him, declared a major in sociology. Now, as a recent college graduate and a diseased father, we interwove our sociological minds one last time.

While Dad was still living, we finished all seven interviews, as planned. I completed drafts of five of the seven chapters, each based on one of the interviews. I also wrote Dad's half of the Introduction based on an earlier conversation we'd had about his work life.

For these five sections and the Introduction, I transcribed some of the words directly from audiotapes but also relied heavily on my notes and memory. I did varying amounts of summarizing and rewording, often significantly rearranging the order of our conversation and always making great efforts to capture the intentions of Dad's original words. In all these cases, he was able to read the drafts, make corrections, and suggest changes.

When Dad died in July, the chapters on Rolling Ridge and Community House Church remained unfinished. In the months since, I transcribed both interviews word for word and then edited them. I stuck as closely as possible to his words, but I had to do substantial editing and rearranging to make the manuscript read easily. I also added some details and made corrections to dates, pulling on other people's memories and resources, including *Faith Road to Rolling Ridge*, a book written in 1990 by Tom Donlon.

In the pages that follow, Nelson Good, my father, reflects on organizations and communities about which he cared deeply. These are his stories, as told to and interpreted by me—his daughter. Thanks to the hours I have spent with his words, the stories have touched and taken up residence in my own.

__Organizing the Book__

Each chapter is split into two parts. I open the chapters in my voice, with sections labeled "Daughter's Voice." These are followed immediately by my dad's reflections, which are written in his voice, based on our interviews, and labeled "Father's Voice."

While Dad was still living, we agreed that if any pieces of our interviews were published, I would clarify that the words attributed to him were *told to and interpreted by* me. The words are not exactly as he would have wanted them, and I would guess that they are, in fact, sometimes altogether wrong. Imperfections aside, I have done my best to tell Dad's stories as accurately and authentically as possible, keeping an ear to the main ideas and general thrust of his words.

Interwoven between the chapters are shorter journal-like entries, written in my voice, telling my personal account of January through July 2005. This book, then, is the story of Dad's reflecting back on his life, while we walked together toward its end.

As I worked on this project in the months and years following Dad's death, alternating my own voice and reflections with his, it felt at times like we were having a conversation—a personal exchange that defied the constraints of time and physical space, a conversation that kept him close to me as I waded in the waters of my grief.

INTRODUCTION

Daughter's Voice
Long After I'm Gone

Wherever they are, most people find comfort in belonging. They create poker clubs and join bowling teams. They go out with co-workers for happy hour. As young adults in Washington, D.C., my parents did not have a bowling team or a favorite bar. Instead, they had supper meetings and discussion groups. One supper group met midweek. A Sunday-night gathering helped found an alternative school called the FLOC Learning Center. Another group eventually developed a retreat center and community called Rolling Ridge. In more recent years, people have continued to gather in my parents' living room—for House Church members meetings, youth activities, and discussions organized for young adults.

Many of the same people were part of several of these different groups, creating an overlapping network of activists who shared similar values and passions. It was from this web that my dad built not only some of his strongest relationships but also his life's work.

In Dad's vision for the world, a dining room table could become a change agent in society. The principal players in the beginnings of Rolling Ridge or House Church did not find one another through an advertisement in the paper. They learned of each other through this network of groups and churches. They gathered together in people's homes around an idea, which, many conversations and work parties later, became—and continue to become—a reality.

As I listened to him talk about his life, I found that over and over Dad was giving intentional thought to creating physical spaces and buildings where people could gather. He and Mom bought houses with large living rooms, which became the sites of many meetings and church gatherings. He helped envision the Rolling Ridge Retreat House, the Thurgood Marshall Center building, and, most recently, a new house for the WSSY/WCSC program. He spoke too of visions for cooperative living arrangements, some still unrealized when he died.

My dad was not a saint nor a celebrity. He knew this about himself. His humility was part of what made him so easy to love. Throughout his life, Dad consciously nurtured the communities to which he belonged. He understood that goodhearted people don't simply decide to up and change the world by themselves. He believed that when we intentionally bring people together, we create the space for ideas to grow, for groups to decide to do radical things—like start schools for troubled kids in inner-city D.C. or retreat centers in mountainous West Virginia—then provide support for each other when things get rough.

And when things got rough, my parents' communities—who by extension became my own—brought us meals, researched alternative treatments, sent countless cards and e-mails, surrounded us with love and desperate prayers. It was a gift that changed me forever.

♣

In writing these opening words, I have wondered what Dad would have had me say. "Make sure they know I was born on a

farm," he might have said. "And that I did my best to love people—with the radical kind of love, the agape kind modeled by
Jesus." Although he rarely spoke so directly about his faith—or
himself—in his life.

In reality, he may also have told you not to bother reading
the chapters of this book, that it was only important for him to
say the words but probably not worth your time to read them.

The pages that follow this introduction leave out large and
crucial pieces of his life—his childhood and family life, to
name two—but they tell something of his vocational path
which was, in many ways, homemade. He was very clear that
these chapters are not comprehensive histories. *They are instead
the story of his personal experience, memory, and analysis of projects
and communities to which he gave much of his time, energy, and
loving care.* They are told through his eyes.

At an event before my dad's funeral, one woman reflected
on "how many structures Nelson built that I now live in." Indeed. Dad sometimes questioned himself for not pursuing a
"career" in the way many of his peers—and his wife—had, but
as you will see in these pages, Dad made his own career of creating structures and medium-sized communities that continue
to house the rest of us.

Father's Voice
Filling the Gap

My career life has been, to some extent, self-made. I didn't
graduate from college with a clear vision for my future. But as
the pieces of my life's work came together, I began to understand that they did all fit into a vision—a larger philosophy of
life that became important to me and then guided my steps.

As a graduate sociology student in the 1970s, I observed a
great need in our society for small and medium-sized community structures. There was a modern tendency toward large-
scale institutions—whether expansive basketball stadiums,

efficient supermarkets, or big schools that were really more like factories. The gap in social structures between these institutions and the nuclear family seemed to me a gaping hole. Extended families were weak. Small neighborhood grocery stores were disappearing. Churches tended to be large and impersonal. In general, "big" and "efficient" were the words of the day.

Without stable, small and medium-sized groups to support them, nuclear families were extremely fragile and vulnerable to breakdown. Where were the intermediate structures—the grocery co-ops, the neighborhood groups, the community soccer leagues—that would give families their "village" in which to raise their children? There were some, but we needed more.

I have come to see my involvement in small community and institutional development as efforts to address society's need for these intermediate social structures. Individuals and families have a hard time making it on their own. They need supportive schools, church communities, and group housing arrangements.

In 1982, Betty, the children, and I took what we called a five-month "sabbatical" from work and city life. By that time, I had already been involved in several groups helping to fill the gap between big and small.[1] During those five months, while we lived as a family in a small cottage at Rolling Ridge in West Virginia, I reflected on where I should invest future energies. Would I continue the work I was doing? Would we as a family continue living in the city? What were my "career" objectives?

It was a clarifying time for me. I recognized that society does need people who can nurture big institutions; they certainly have their place. But I did not think they were my place. My gifts would be better suited in developing and nurturing smaller institutions. I still felt called to smaller projects, and I would continue to focus my skills and energy in that direction.

Here, in these pages, I tell some of my story. It is the story of a Lancaster County farm boy who found his way to the city of

Washington, D.C., and then stayed for almost forty years. These are the stories—through my eyes—of the small and medium-sized communities and projects in which I have been involved in my adult years, combined with my reflections on their strengths and flaws.

Whether through paid work or informal commitments, Betty and I sought to develop and nurture groups and communities that then supported and surrounded us as we raised our children. Today, after a short fight with cancer, I am approaching the end of my life at sixty-one. I will die surrounded by my immediate family and, beyond them, circles of love wider and stronger than I could have imagined. Many will say I have given much, but the truth is I have received, in return, far more than the worth of my weight in gold.

Long After
I'm Gone

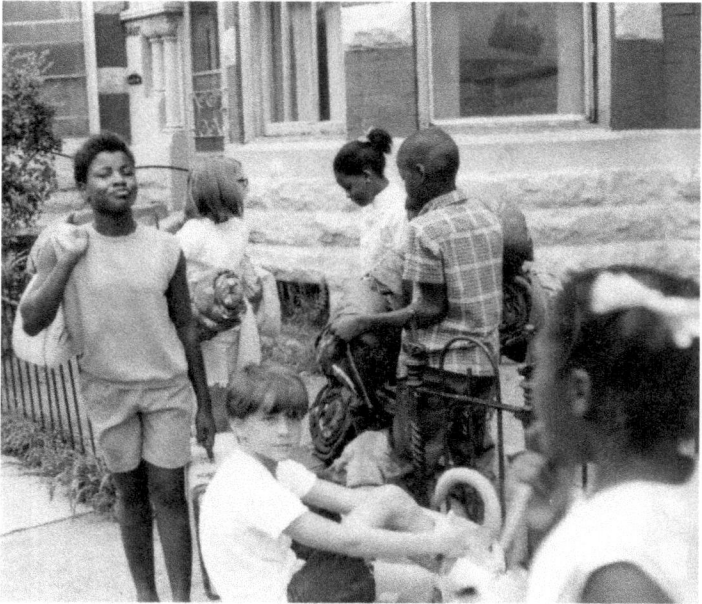

Children from W Street participated in a variety of Friendship Flat activities, including trips to the country. Photographer unknown

Chapter 1

FRIENDSHIP FLAT

Daughter's Voice
At Home?

The April 9 assassination of Martin Luther King Jr. brought riots and fires to Washington's streets, just blocks from the volunteer house where my parents would move in September.

> *I wish I could have been here in 1968*
> *to see you, Lancaster County farm boy,*
> *plopped into the colorful tumult of Washington, D.C.*

Friendship Flat was a youth community center on W Street in northwest Washington. The center was begun in 1966 by Bob and Esther Wert as a project of the Mennonite Church[2] and was staffed by volunteers who lived on the two floors above it. Between 1968 and 1970, my parents spent the first two years of their married life living there with four other volunteers.

I picture Dad standing at an upstairs window in the house. His gray corduroys are starting to wear at the knees—something he hadn't noticed until his wife mentioned it to him the night before. He hooks his right thumb into a belt loop as though it is anchoring him firmly to the floor.

In his left hand, a mug steams with cheap coffee. He will never kick the habit and years later will keep doughnuts in the freezer, warming them to cut the bitterness of the dark liquid.

The paisley shirt sprawled on a nearby chair is his, but he stands with only a white undershirt; a hole is forming in the one armpit. His blue eyes look out through dark-rimmed glasses and, at first glance, it is impossible to tell if he is closer to laughing or sighing.

Below, he sees more than the pavement of W Street. He sees a river of pain, power struggles, and racism flowing between homes and cars, past white volunteers and black neighbors, down the block—and he understands that he's swimming in it.

> *What would you have said then*
> *had you known you'd still be here*
> *more than thirty years later,*
> *hunching down in front of the television*
> *every Sunday for the Skins game,*
> *passing bundled men by the sidewalk*
> *on your way to the bank,*
> *and making sure every door and window is locked*
> *before you go to bed at night?*

It was Christmas 2001. I had decided to write poems for my family. I wrote one for Dad: "Outsider." I realize now the poem's title had more to do with me than him; I grew up straddling the white, Mennonite world of summer church camp, and the mostly black world of city buses and public schools. My skin felt like it was glowing. I didn't quite belong anywhere.

I assumed Dad would have felt the same way, working so closely with African-Americans one day, and mingling among coverings and plain coats at his father's Lancaster County funeral the next. But he read the poem and said he never thought of himself like that—as an outsider. Last year, I finally revised the poem and re-titled it "At Home."

You smirk, just a little and never harshly,
at the countless dreamers
who pass through this place in their twenties
with visions of changing the world
but move out before they hit thirty
and go on to drive BMW's, invest in stock,
and live in seas of caucasianality.

One could say my dad was a serious man, but this would be dreadfully incomplete. Dad's humor was often subtle, like the wrinkle that appeared in the space between his forehead and his eyes. Mom, more than anyone, could not tell when he was joking. "But don't you see his crease?" her friends would ask.

He was an artist when it came to leadership. He spent his life setting people at ease with a joke—in difficult conversations, student seminars, board meetings, staff meetings, church meetings, meetings, meetings, and more meetings.

Still, serious or not, Dad did build, work, and befriend with thoughtful intention. He was a realist and made all his decisions very carefully, never on a whim. I still cannot leave my Philadelphia home on a dark, urban night without his voice in my head. "Never take unnecessary risks," he liked to remind me. "Never take unnecessary risks."

I also can't look at the basketball hoop hanging in the alley behind our house in D.C. without thinking about Dad and his head full of risk-calculation. Ever since he built the backboard out of old floorboards and braced it to our garage roof, he insisted that we keep it locked up between games. This involves wrapping a chain diagonally across the rim and locking it in place with a padlock, so no basketball can fit through.

"Dad, I don't understand why we have to keep the hoop locked," I remember insisting. "It seems so selfish. Why do you act like we're better than other people?" I was an adolescent with answers. I also went to school with kids in the neighborhood who knew about the chain, and I was embarrassed.

"Have you seen what happened to other hoops in the neighborhood? How long have they lasted?" Dad would respond impatiently. We had had this conversation before. He went on to list them: the hoop down the alley that was there about a month when it got dunked on and broken. Another one that drew so many complaints from neighbors, they had to take it down. "If we leave our hoop unlocked," he continued, "and kids start hanging out in our alley, making noise, maybe even bringing drugs."

That was a complete sentence, because I could guess how it ended. The neighbors would complain, the cops might get involved, we'd have to take the hoop down, and then we would never be able to play basketball in our alley again.

"I still think it's selfish," I said again, stubbornly, and turned to go upstairs.

"Deborah, I didn't move to the city yesterday." Apparently he wasn't done. "I have spent years in the inner city, and trying to create safe places for fun to happen. It's not that I don't care. It's that I do, and I understand how these things work."

I am not convinced that Dad's answers were all exactly right, but he always had a thorough explanation for why he did what he did. And he was convinced it was this intentionality and moderation that kept him in the city year after year—nearly forty in all.

But you have stayed,
long enough to call this home.
long enough that when you speak,
today's young dreamers listen,
as though wisdom were oozing thickly
from your ears and off your tongue,
long enough that
when you step into Ben's Chili Bowl on U Street
the owner knows who you are,
and when you walk the streets of your city,

cab-driver hat on your head
and worn briefcase in your hand,
people can tell you belong here
because your feet fall comfortably
with each step.

My mom recently drove me and my brother Jason through the neighborhood where Friendship Flat opened its doors to children and teens from 1966 to 1973. She pointed out the brick row house at 1425 W Street and talked about how intimidating the neighborhood had felt when they first moved in. She had grown up in Ethiopia, the daughter of missionaries, and Dad on a farm. The W Street community was a foreign land. As newlyweds two or three years younger than I, and as outsiders, they floundered to root Friendship Flat in this urban, African-American neighborhood and negotiated many daunting social realities for the first time.

I looked out the car window at the old wood of what was once Friendship Flat's side porch and imagined kids sitting on its railings and steps. Today, as in many urban communities, this neighborhood is changing and gentrifying. New construction is going up where a drug market once thrived. Rising prices are forcing out those who can't afford their rent or property taxes, and a new population is moving in—the ongoing urban dilemma.

The funny thing about Dad was that, even after thirty years in the city, you would never doubt that he grew up a Mennonite in Lancaster County. I still wonder at all the years Dad spent working with people so different from him, who were no doubt amused by his slower, country ways, his lolling voice and slight Pennsylvania Dutch accent.

The rural landscape of his childhood was scarred by farming accidents, by lives and fingers lost, by near misses and sorrows. But, Dad told us with some sense of pride, Grandpa had raised seven boys on a farm with such careful thought that no one had ever been seriously injured. Like father, like son, I suppose.

♣

I was twenty-two years old when George W. Bush became serious about his threat to invade Iraq. Crowds of people filled the streets of D.C., where I was living at the time as a recent college graduate. *This is what democracy looks like! This is what democracy looks like!* The chants practically ran through my dreams.

On a biting day in January, I joined a large group organized for civil disobedience—the practice of risking arrest, refusing to obey a government's laws when that government is viewed as being unjust. We marched to H Street, in front of the White House, and sat down. We carried signs and pictures of Martin Luther King Jr., a day before our country was celebrating his birthday. Cops ordered us to move, dragged us to the sidewalk, stared us down, arrested no one. We locked arms, sat down again.

Our supporters stood legally on the sidewalk to witness the confrontation, and my dad, looking gray-haired and conservative between dreadlocks and nose rings, was among them. *This is what democracy looks like! This is what democracy looks like!*

When it became clear that the police had no intentions of arresting us, we decided to leave the street and march back to a nearby park. Drummers played. Some folks struck up a song, and someone led us in a neo-pagan "spiral dance." We held hands and moved as a line, winding toward the center of the circle, out again, around and around.

I looked across that circle and saw Dad, long hair to his left, long skirt to his right. It was the only time I remember Dad dancing. And I realized: This was a man adept at adapting, open and accepting, a man who had spent his life moving between cultures, while somehow always holding his own.

You carry the city in your hands,
the farm in your feet;
and all life's paradox in between.
And somehow, wherever you find yourself,
wherever you are,
you invite others to feel as you do:
always,
always,
at home.

Father's Voice
Mennonites on W Street

When I was graduating from college in 1968, most young men were immediately drafted for Vietnam. As a Mennonite and a pacifist, I would not participate in war, choosing instead to seek a term of "1W Service"—an alternative for conscientious objectors.

While still a senior at Eastern Mennonite College (EMC), I began looking for a two-year volunteer placement that would fulfill my enlistment requirement. Betty and I were engaged at the time. A Mennonite voluntary service organization offered us a placement in Haiti or in Washington, D.C.[3] We chose the latter.

Even though I was born and raised on a dairy farm, I was drawn to the city during college, where I studied urban sociology. The Civil Rights Movement was making the news. As the movement's focus shifted from the South to the northern cities, it brought to light a different kind of segregation. White flight to the suburbs was leaving behind pockets of poverty where low-income, African-American communities were depleted of resources. Without the tax base of wealthier families, inner-city schools, libraries, and social services were far from adequate. As a result, cities were places of ferment—and social activism, as people cried out for change.

I wanted to connect with the plight and energy of the city. My interest in urban studies had taken me to New York City in 1967 for a brief summer seminar with about a dozen other college students. Now it was taking me and Betty to Washington, D.C. We were married on August 18, 1968, and after a short honeymoon at a cottage in the mountains, we moved to a community center on W Street for two years of voluntary service.

__ Our Assignment __

In 1966, Bob and Esther Wert helped found Friendship Flat in northwest Washington, at 14th and W Streets, on a block made up of row houses and walk-up apartment buildings. Friendship Flat was a row house with volunteers living on its two upper floors. The first floor and the basement served as a drop-in center for children and youth. When Betty and I arrived, the project was only two years old and still becoming established in the neighborhood.

I was to be the coordinator for our group of six volunteers, managing finances and providing logistical and emotional support. As a unit, we focused most of our energy and attention on planning and leading youth and children's activities. Some of the volunteers also had part-time jobs elsewhere in the city. Betty, for one, volunteered in the guidance counseling office at a nearby public high school.

Our weeks had a basic rhythm to them. On Monday, Wednesday, and Friday, we opened the center immediately after school for club activities: tutoring, arts and crafts, and shop. The center was open later in the evening for recreation. A pool table kept kids busy in one room, a ping pong table in another room, and a third room had table games. On Sunday afternoons, we offered Bible classes.

Thursdays we set aside as our "unit day." The six of us tried not to make other commitments, reserving the day to spend time together. Our days kept us up late; we usually did not eat supper until after we closed the youth center at nine o'clock, so we grew weary. Even though we weren't leading youth activities all the time, the experience of living on the block and building many informal relationships with adults as well as kids in the neighborhood took a lot of energy.

I remember how stressful it was. It was intensely cross-cultural for me—for all of us. We were outsiders, the only white faces on the block, and many of us came from rural and small-town backgrounds. Sometimes on Thursdays, we took excursions out of D.C., away from the intensity of the city. Our "unit day" helped renew our energy and preserve the relationships within the group.

Beyond the weekly activities at the center, we sometimes used our unit van to take small groups of kids on field trips: bike rides, hikes, canoe trips. I also remember volunteers taking families from the neighborhood on day trips to farms. Once, we took a group to my family farm in Lancaster County, Pennsylvania. It was fascinating for many of the families to get outside the city—to see cows and calves, walk along the creek, and touch grass. Betty remembers how frightened a toddler became when his mother tried to set him down on the grass. It was something foreign to him.

During the summer, we also took kids to Black Rock, a Mennonite camp in Pennsylvania. At Black Rock, a few weeks every summer were geared for inner-city youth, so we would drive groups up to the camp and then stay for the week as counselors.

__*Memories*__

Even amid stress and imperfections, our two years on W Street brought about positive relationships and valuable memories. I probably learned and grew as much from the experience as any of the children on the block.

I expect we were far more naïve than we realized. I remember clearly one day during our first year when I took a group of kids to a public swimming pool at Cardoza High School. During the swimming activity, I accidentally jabbed one of the kids in his eye with my finger. He wasn't hurt badly, but it was sore. Afterwards, I did not let it enter my mind that I should go with this eleven-year-old back to his mother to explain what had happened. He lived in a walk-up apartment building. An apartment building like that was the kind of place I had been taught—probably unconsciously—to fear. It intimidated me, especially after dark. So the boy went home alone.

Later, I got a phone call from his mother, a widow with ten children whose husband had died falling off a trash truck. She told me that this was no way for an adult to handle such a situation. Experiences like that let me know I was still learning what it meant to be a responsible person.

I will always remember, too, the day Betty and I took her girls' club—maybe six girls eleven through fourteen years old—to the C&O Canal. There was a place where we rented bikes to ride on the towpath, alongside the canal. We set off. Betty was at the front of the string of bikes, and I was bringing up the rear. Up ahead, one girl was swatting at a gnat and lost control of her bike. Betty remembers hearing a shriek, and then turning to discover that Betty Reeves had vanished from view—girl and bike together! She had plunged right off the towpath into the canal. The bike sank about six feet to the bottom, but fortunately Betty Reeves clung to weeds at the side of the canal. I don't care to know whether or not she knew how to swim.

By this point, the whole string of girls had stopped and gathered around. I got off my bike, went down to the water as fast as I could, and managed to pull young Betty out of the water and up to the path, soaked. But the bike was nowhere to be seen. Before long, I was in the canal up to my neck, treading water, feeling around with my toe for the lost bicycle. I found it, hooked it with my foot, and hoisted it up to where I could grab it with my hand. Somehow—don't ask me how—I managed to maneuver myself to the side of the canal, where Betty and the girls helped pull me and the bike, both dripping wet, out of the water.

When we got home that night, Betty went with Betty Reeves to talk with her mother and explain what had happened. We had learned from my experience that this was, of course, what a responsible adult should do to build trust in a community. Betty was very apologetic and remembers Mrs. Reeves accepting her apology.

We have learned since that many of the girls in that girls' club, including Betty Reeves, did not make it. They lost their lives to AIDS, drug violence, or other difficulties common to high-risk city neighborhoods.

Another memory: One weekend, two of the volunteers had taken a team of the older youth to Pennsylvania to play basketball against some Mennonite young people. We did not allow some of the kids to go on the trip because they were too young or because of their behavior. That weekend, it snowed three to four inches. A group of those who weren't on the trip showed up at our door and asked me to open the recreation center for them. They knew I was the principal of sorts, the guy in charge (I believe they called me "Mister Nelson").

But the recreation center was not open Saturday evenings, and I would not open it for them. They became very belligerent and started throwing snowballs at our windows. The snowballs broke the panes in the first-floor bay window. What was I going to do with these kids?

Instead of acting out of my anger, I went out on the street and started throwing snowballs back at them. We got into quite a snowball battle. I chased them down to the park and even caught some of them and washed their faces in the snow. It was a way to divert their energy into fun instead of destruction. I think they were very impressed that I would take them on. Afterward, they agreed to come in and clean up the glass, while I boarded up the windowpanes.

__*What We Wanted*__

As volunteers at Friendship Flat, we understood ourselves to be visitors in the neighborhood, especially because most of us were merely passing through. Transitional leadership, we knew, made our efforts unsustainable, and I wanted to create a community organization—a neighborhood council—to encourage leadership and a sense of ownership within the neighborhood itself.

One such effort was to create a mothers' club among the women in the neighborhood. It was hard to coordinate and did not last. But we did take one wonderful trip. A number of adults in the community joined us in planning a neighborhood field trip to Luray Caverns. With summer funding from the city, we rented a chartered bus and piled onboard—a whole crowd of children and moms and, if I remember correctly, one father. We have a picture of the group posing in the Caverns, full of smiles. You can easily pick out the Mennonite volunteers—me, Betty, Eva Beidler—in our white skin and dark-rimmed glasses. Everyone had a marvelous time, and many felt really good about the roles they had in planning the trip.

The Luray Caverns trip was one glimpse of the kind of work I wanted to do: cooperative and empowering of the neighborhood. But during our time on W Street, glimpses were as good as we got. Creating more of a lasting foundation, a community organization with internal leadership, proved very difficult as we were outsiders bringing our idea of "healthy community" to families who had lived there and would continue living there far longer than we would. We were an intrusion, unconnected to any existing institution, like a local church or school, and we were transient. Our efforts, for the most part, floundered.

__*A Flawed Project?*__

Last year, we had a reunion of former Friendship Flat volunteers (maybe fifteen to twenty folks), and nearly twice as

many who had grown up on W Street and remembered coming
to Friendship Flat as kids between 1966 and 1973. We were all
thirty years older and had a marvelous time sharing memories
and catching up.

A number of those who had been children or youth on W
Street expressed how much they had loved Friendship Flat. It
was a wonderful place, they said. They recalled many positive
experiences that inspired them to develop and grow. More importantly, the caring relationships cultivated at the center
helped them feel valued and included, significantly shaping
their young lives.

Indeed, many of our efforts in the neighborhood were positive; we had as many as 125 children and youth involved in our
activities in one way or another. But as time went on, I had
more and more questions about the larger effects of the "good"
we were doing.

Children who participated in the Fresh Air program, for
example, had a great time. The program matched city kids up
with farm families, who would host them in the country for
two weeks at a time. The farm families had money and big
hearts. In their efforts to host the inner-city children, the families showered the kids with gifts and goodies and attention.
We would sometimes observe how hard it was for the children
to then return to city streets, where they had to fend for themselves, and to homes that were broken by poverty and hardship.

To make things worse, the Fresh Air families were white.
And so were we. For many of the children living in the inner
city in 1968, "black" meant poverty while "white" meant opportunity, money, and kindness. I felt that the fact that we were
an all-white household in an all-black neighborhood, providing kids with special opportunities and relationships, reinforced racist stereotypes.

There were other structural problems, too. Friendship Flat
created a sense of dependency in some kids on the block, a

problem made worse because we were so transient—most of us did not stay on the block for more than two years.

A number of volunteers developed informal friendships with neighborhood youth. The kids would stop by the house for help with schoolwork or just to hang out. Once, I remember a volunteer teaching a sixteen-year-old how to drive so he could get his license. These one-on-one relationships were crucial. Many of the children did not have significant dependable relationships in their lives and needed adults they could trust.

But sometimes they became very attached to the volunteers and then were let down, yet again, when each of us eventually left the street after our terms of service. Even though we were aware of it and tried to be cautious, over-dependency remained a tendency inherent in our short-term service model.

It was hard for me to clearly legitimize our being there. I imagined the larger neighborhood looking in on us. Why were these six young people coming in here? What was their purpose? Unlike an institution providing a clear service—like a school or a clinic—Friendship Flat was very informal. Yes, we provided nice activities, but who said the neighborhood wanted those activities in the first place?

As I understood it, one of the Mennonite church's objectives in founding the youth center was that our presence on the block, and our Bible classes, would eventually be the seeds for developing an inner-city church. I was very cautious about the idea. I had reservations about the institutional church to begin with. Then the proposal that we white folks would start a church in an African-American neighborhood, without any connections to existing community structures, seemed not only difficult but questionable from a perspective of racial consciousness. Besides, many of the families on the block already had church connections. No doubt these are the reasons Friendship Flat never became an urban church.

Many of us volunteers were critical of the institutional church, generally, for accommodating to the racism of U.S. society, and for drawing lines between those who were "Christian" and those who were not.

I observed how people I sometimes met in the city—people who did not necessarily attend church or talk about Jesus—better exemplified the radical love of Christ than some I knew who were at church every Sunday morning. These were committed people who gave of themselves willingly in addressing the needs of their communities. Did the church have the right to decide what language and rituals were required for entrance into the kingdom of heaven? As time went on, I came to believe that the kingdom is often present where you least expect it.

After our two years as volunteers, Betty and I moved to a nearby apartment building. For the next six years, I worked as the (paid) half-time administrator for Friendship Flat and one other Mennonite voluntary service unit in Washington. I continued to question the legitimacy of the W Street project. While Friendship Flat provided volunteers with a remarkable experience, and while it did succeed in creating a place of connection and support in a troubled area of the city, the overall model did not lead to broader structural change, and in some ways, I felt, perpetuated the problems of the inner city. There were other challenges as well, and in 1973, the Mennonite church closed Friendship Flat at my recommendation.[4]

january 30, 2005

Last Wednesday, the twenty-sixth, was perhaps the longest day of my life. It was five of four in the afternoon. Dad lay on a stretcher in the hallway outside the emergency room at Washington Hospital Center, preparing himself for the possibility that the serious pain in his back would require surgery.

Mom was taking a much-needed nap at home; we had spent the previous night taking shifts in the ER waiting room. And I was literally minutes from leaving Dad's side for the train station when Doctor Noel walked up. She was a petite, brown-skinned woman with kind eyes and long silver earrings (for some reason, I remember the earrings). I was already in danger of missing my train, hoping to return to Philadelphia after what had turned into a very long weekend in D.C.

Then Doctor Noel, oh so gently, dropped on us the ton of bricks that she was carrying. The CT-scan. The baseball-sized mass. The word *malignant*. I wonder now what it was like to be her. How did it feel to meet with two unsuspecting strangers and hand them a bomb?

A few minutes later, she delivered the news over the phone to my mom, who had recently awakened from her nap.

Dad reached up for me. I'm sure it was at least another fifteen minutes before I fully realized what the doctor had said, but I hugged him anyway.

He immediately thought of Mom sitting at home alone, the phone ringing, the doctor's voice on the other end. Who could go be with her? Who could drive her to the hospital? Grace, we decided. Grace who had been a good friend for years, who had helped raise me and my brothers and lived in the neighborhood.

I called Mom until she picked up. It was clear she had not yet computed the doctor's words either. Other than a twinge of panic, her voice was calm, relaxed even. I handed my cell phone to Dad.

Then I turned and shared the news with Dan, a family friend who—if this isn't serendipity, I don't know what is—had just arrived (he was to take my place at the hospital after I left for the train). He nodded his head, up down, up down. He said he would call Grace. Then I did not leave the hospital, did not catch my train and was not to return to Philadelphia, in fact, for weeks.

That night, I stayed at the hospital and hardly slept. My head hurt, a constant, dull ache. Whereas Dad rested (somewhat) with the aid of potent pain medication, the nurses' station could not even give me a Tylenol unless I was admitted. This—the irony of it—was the funniest part of my day; I may have even laughed. They gave me orange juice instead of medication.

Today, four days later, my eyes hurt from all the tears and lack of sleep. The whole family is here now: Ryan and Hannah from Indiana, Jason and Bryn from Virginia. It feels like a death sentence. And part of all of us knows that it probably is. What do you do with such a thing?

They say everyone copes differently. Apparently one of my coping mechanisms is to busy myself with practical details. I call my uncle with the day's update. I e-mail a church friend who has offered to coordinate our meals, the first of which awaited us at home last night: homemade bread and jam, rice, and chicken curry—enough to feed a small congregation—from Eva Beidler. I shovel the snow off our back steps and sort the mail.

It feels good to do something. Maybe it's my attempt to create order when all else is out of my control. I wonder if it looks like I'm on top of things. Really, I am breaking.

I cope, too, by plugging myself into the sprawling people-web that surrounds us. Every night, I check e-mail—my parents' and my own. "You are in our thoughts constantly," writes one friend. "Has anyone offered to help with laundry yet?" writes another. "Do you have a field we could plow? A barn we could build?"

Lesson of the moment: I am not a little autonomous being, deciding this and that about my own life without interference. I am a thread in a tapestry of people. Should I ever forget my interconnectedness with the world, I will be lost.

In seventh grade, Mr. Hughes, my homeroom teacher, succeeded in making an impression on all of us who sat before him, intimidated by our first day of junior high school. "You're all going to die someday," he told us. Indeed we will. The difference between me and my dad, then, is that he has a better idea how he might go.

Dad says death is not something he's thought enough about. Perhaps most of us could say the same. And tonight, I consider writing about death—as an idea, a scientific process, a theological concept—but I find myself wanting to write instead about mystery.

"When death comes," writes Mary Oliver in her poem with that title, "like the hungry bear in autumn; /. . . . / I want to step through the door full of curiosity, wondering: / what is it going to be like, that cottage of darkness?" (1-2, 9-10)

When we each breathe our last, I have to say, honestly, I really don't know what happens. Clouds and angels? Eternal inner peace? Absolutely nothing?

I happily allow others their certainties about the after-life—heaven, hell, neither, both, something else altogether. I prefer living with the mystery of it all, with Oliver's almost childlike curiosity about what will be there, on the other side of that passage.

Before, thoughts like these wandered through my mind on occasion—monthly perhaps. Now they enter the routine mulling of my days. I feel I have moved into a new room of this sprawling farmhouse called life, and there's no turning back.

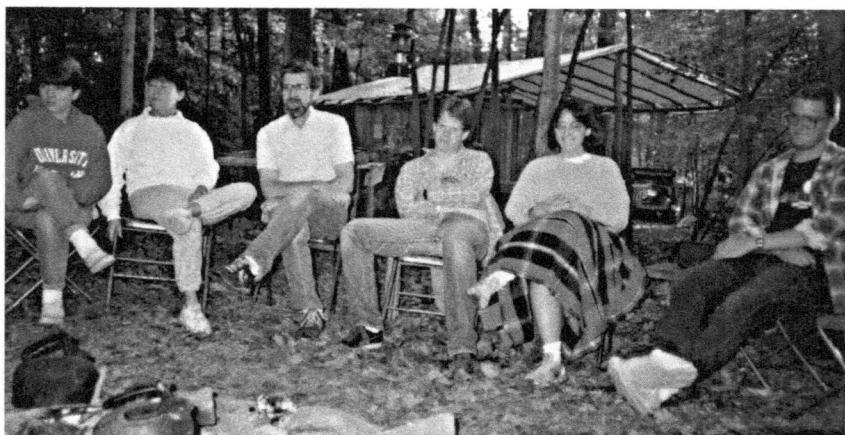

As one of WSSY's co-directors, Nelson led students in seminar discussions and took the groups on camping trips. Photo credit: Doug Hertzler

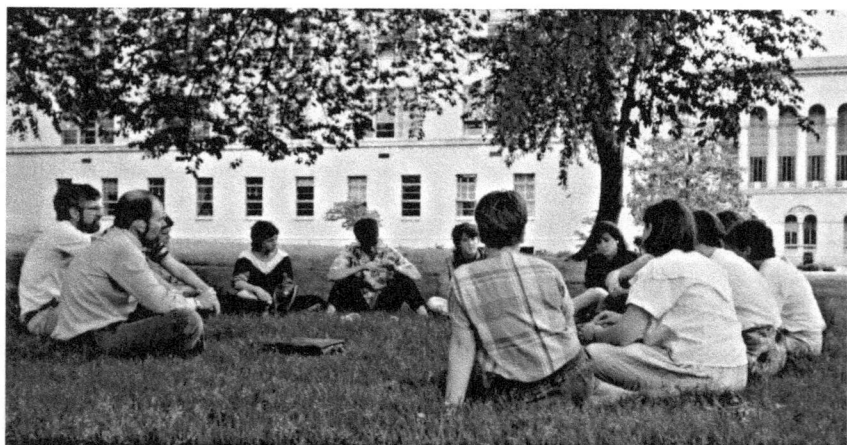

Chapter 2

WASHINGTON STUDY-SERVICE YEAR

Daughter's Voice
The Servant Leader

Mom's hands were wrist deep in dish-washing vigor when Dad came running down the stairs. Or maybe they weren't. She can't remember that part for sure. What she does remember, clear as day, was the excitement in his voice when he told her what he had just learned from a phone call: "I think it's really going to happen!"

Dad was not one to exclaim about anything. His most common answer to any of a number of questions—about his day or his job or his summer vacation—was one word, with a period at the end. *Fine.* This was mostly, I think, his modesty talking. He did not speak excitedly about himself and usually preferred to ask you about your life anyway.

But on this particular day, Dad had something to say worth an exclamation point. He had finally received approval from Eastern Mennonite College (EMC) for a small brainstorm of a program, an idea that blossomed out of his critique of Friendship Flat. The new program for college students, soon named

Washington Study-Service Year (WSSY), would open that fall, with Dad as its first coordinator. The year was 1976.

Six years earlier, after serving for two as volunteers at Friendship Flat, my parents had moved one block away into a sixth-floor apartment—still a young married couple—living on their own for the first time. They both started graduate school at Catholic University, Mom in social work, Dad in sociology. Dad juggled two courses a semester alongside his half-time position as administrator of D.C.'s Mennonite voluntary service units and a part-time taxi-driving job.

Dad did not have a clear vision for the path his future would take. His life had a way of unfolding, sometimes with painstaking effort, the way it takes care and patience to open the convoluted folds of a travel map. And though he sometimes criticized himself for lacking career direction, I believe he learned to trust and thrive in this unfolding process.

The WSSY program's beginning was one un-fold in Dad's travel map. This was the first of several times in his life when Dad helped plant and grow an idea, and in so doing, created a job and found someone to pay him to do it. When he died almost thirty years later, Dad had never undertaken a traditional job search nor written a resume.

I have been floundering in my twenties, entirely undecided about what to do with my life. On a camping trip the year after Dad's death, I sat around a campfire and polled five of my friends about my future career direction. Counselor or social worker? I asked. Graphic artist? Editor? Carpenter?

"You're like your dad," they informed me. "You won't have one career; you'll get involved in different projects; you'll create work for yourself."

I'm always flattered to be compared with my father, but this was not entirely good news. I have longed for one career—for the routine of it, the health insurance. Yet there is something inspiring about Dad's story. In so many ways, he was just an ordinary guy, one who believed in himself enough to take his ideas somewhere—to talk, propose, sweat, and breathe them into being.

"It sometimes amazes me how this all came to be," he told me, speaking of WSSY. "Clearly, the birth of WSSY was a creative process. I was a networker. The program came about because of relationships and conversations with people, not because of long, well-written documents." This is all true, but WSSY also came to be because my dad had persistence and what I call *staying power*, in an age when most of us can't pay attention long enough to hand-write a letter before we have to stop and check our e-mail.

♣

In designing WSSY, Dad hoped to avoid some of the problems he had found so troubling at Friendship Flat. The WSSY program would bring college students to D.C. for a year of "experiential education." Instead of serving as the volunteer staff of a community center, Dad's vision had WSSY students plugging into established organizations as interns. They would come to the city to offer their skills and help, but more importantly, to observe and to learn.

Janet Liechty, a former WSSY student speaking at Dad's funeral, described the program. "Here was a program that didn't lecture to you," she said. "It created spaces for your voice—and others'—to be heard. It didn't analyze the world for you; it put you in the world and asked you to reflect on what you experienced, processing it within the community. It didn't emphasize ratings and grades but drew us into learning for its own sake."[5]

Spaces for your voice. Within the community. Learning for its own sake. I think Dad would have liked those words. Dad saw WSSY as an alternative to the spoon-feeding that sometimes happens in classroom settings. "Real students," he told me, "should be able to think for themselves."

I think, to Dad, *experiential education* was not just a WSSY catch phrase. It was a concept that described his own father. Ira

Mathias Good, a farmer with an eighth-grade education, was far wiser than some people who decorate their offices with degrees.

I see now that Grandpa Good taught my dad to be a student of life, and in turn, Dad showed his students how to observe and engage their surroundings, to read their lives as one might read a book, taking notes and jotting questions in the margins. *What is it like to be a racial minority? I think I feel more self-conscious . . . and why are D.C. neighborhoods still so segregated after Desegregation? Maybe "white flight" has something to do with it. . . . How should I respond to beggars on the street? How can this city's huge institutions be changed for the better? And where—amid all this neglect and hardship—is God?*

♣

A large manila envelope recently arrived in the mail from my mom. I carefully pulled out two booklets, faded and tearing at their stapled binding. I was surprised how small they were; both together could easily slide under my bedroom door. Yet on these two flimsy booklets, Dad built not only WSSY but also much of his life.

The brick-red one is titled *The Servant as Leader,* and the light blue, *The Institution as Servant.* They were written by Robert Greenleaf and published in 1970 and 1972 respectively. "Ours are revolutionary times," writes Greenleaf on page 2 of the first. "Not so much for the extent of turbulence and disruption as because of the emergence of a significant number of thoughtful and aware people who see more clearly the world as it is and are not satisfied with it."

Becoming a servant leader, he says, "requires that the concerned individual accept the problems he sees in the world as his own personal task, as a means of achieving his own integrity."[6]

I asked Mom recently what she thought servant leadership meant to Dad. It meant, she said, that he wanted what was good for others. He took it upon himself to bring others' strengths to light while not calling attention to his own.

Servanthood was a popular idea in my Mennonite upbringing. My dad loved this idea, but it has not always been a comfortable one for me. Theologically speaking, the word meant that we were to deny ourselves, as Christ denied himself on the cross, for the betterment of others. Among Mennonite women in particular, this was often combined with submissiveness and self-sacrifice. As I grew older, I became conscious of all the possibilities and pleasures women gave up in the name of "servanthood," and the word soured in my mouth.

But in his writing, Robert Greenleaf intertwines *servant* with *leader*. His response to my qualms about service? "The true servant," he writes, "must *lead* to be a complete [person]!"[7] The sentence is underlined heavily by Dad's pencil.

Dad saw Greenleaf's writing as providing an alternative to the shouts of many young radicals in the '60s and '70s who believed existing institutions should be torn apart, leveled, destroyed. In the small, light blue book, Greenleaf observes that "until recently, caring was largely man-to-man, [but] now most of it is mediated through institutions—often large, complex, powerful, impersonal; not always competent; sometimes corrupt."[8] He argues that to build a better society, major institutions must develop the capacity to serve. Institutions must themselves be servants.

Dad hoped to teach his WSSY students that institutions are a necessary part of a productive society. Instead of working to tear them down, we should work with existing institutions—churches, schools, businesses, and nonprofits—to generate new leadership and board structures that serve others rather than protect themselves.

Yet, as Janet said at his funeral, Dad did not believe in servant institutions as an end themselves. He saw them merely as "the scaffolding for something real to happen."[9]

♣

One Sunday morning nearly a year after Dad's death, I led worship at West Philadelphia Mennonite Fellowship, where I have made attempts at being present and part of things. After the service, a young man approached me. His hair was sandy-blonde, framing his face with a full beard. He looked familiar, though I couldn't place him exactly. Josh, he said, was his name. Because of something I had said during the morning's service, he'd pieced together part of my family tree.

"I want to tell you that I knew your father," Josh said. It was one of those moments when everything else in the room fades into dull noise. I zeroed in.

"You were a Sojourners intern, weren't you?" I asked, realizing why I recognized him. *Sojourners* is a magazine with offices close to my childhood home. "You're the tree guy." He smiled. Yes, he was the tree guy, the one who had climbed one of the poplars next to my parents' house in D.C. and took it down, limb by limb.

"I did quite a bit of work for your dad, both in trees near your house in D.C. and out at Rolling Ridge.[10] I only had a few conversations with your dad, but one of them turned out to be crucial to me."

Go on.

"We were driving in his car one day, and I told him I had dropped out of high school when I was seventeen." Dad was a high school dropout, too—at sixteen to help on the farm he was to inherit from his father. I sometimes wonder how different my life would be had he opted to stay on the farm instead of leaving for college where he developed a fascination for cities.

Josh continued. "He explained that he took his GED and went back to get a Bachelors, then a Masters." He paused thoughtfully. "Your dad encouraged me to think that I could, in fact, go back and continue my education."

Later, Josh followed up with an e-mail. *it was an important conversation for me. one of a few pivotal ones that led me back to school at 28.* Josh is now studying at a university near Philadelphia.

i first met your dad on his tractor at rolling ridge, he wrote. *i liked him because he was on a tractor and had a beard and was quiet and kind.* I was at a coffee shop with my laptop when I read his e-mail. I felt that familiar warm burning in my eyes. *your dad was a sweet, humble, and encouraging man.*

This humility was part of what servant leadership meant to him: Instead of building structures for his own self-aggrandizement, Dad created environments where other people's gifts could be cultivated, used, and recognized. The best test of the servant leader, writes Robert Greenleaf, is this: "Do those served grow as persons; do they become healthier, wiser, freer, more autonomous while being served?"[11]

At one point, when I was interviewing Dad about WSSY, he commented that students seemed to hold him in high regard. "Though I couldn't tell you why," he said. When listening to the recording later, I shook my head, laughing. This was classic Dad: dousing his own self-compliment with a bucket of humility.

Students liked Dad because he believed in them. "Show interest," Ira Good, Dad's father, would tell his boys again and again. Showing interest in students' lives became one of Dad's key assets as WSSY's first coordinator. The job—one he kept for more than a decade—gave him the opportunity to do some of what he did best, even though he had no counseling or clinical license to prove it: He listened well, accepted others without judgment; he offered them vast spaces for growth and undue amounts of trust. This is why, when his own kids were learning to drive, Dad would lead us out into the frantic bustle of the D.C. beltway, trusting us to handle the heavy and aggressive traffic, while Mom sat in the back seat, a pillow pressed to her face.

Dad believed everyone was "special," a word he often used to describe others, including me. When my battles with self-doubt clamor loudly in my head, it is still the memory of Dad's soothing affirmation that calms them. This, more than anything, was his secret to working with young adults, many of us sloshing around in our shabby attempts to believe in ourselves.

Starting the WSSY program was not simple. As Dad makes clear in his telling of the story, a number of people helped key pieces fall into place—from acquiring the building to convincing Eastern Mennonite College his proposal was worth their attention. Once it got rolling, Dad served as the program's coordinator for its first eleven years, always with an assistant coordinator working by his side. Later, he became involved again as a board member and then as the brains and vision behind the program's search for a new facility.[12]

Changes to the WSSY program over the years have been met with voices of both support and resistance. Surely Dad felt some sense of loss with each significant transition: the decision to give students a one-semester option, to rename the program, and to move from the old stucco house on South Dakota Avenue. Yet Dad also understood that the survival of institutions sometimes requires a letting go of the answers of the past, a willingness to change, and an openness to what will become.

Father's Voice
Breaking Out of the Classroom

$$\_\_\textit{The Idea}\_\_$$

As with most things I've been involved in, the program that came to be called "Wissy" began as an idea. And as the little idea developed, several people—some unwittingly—became key in bringing the thing to reality. Gerry Meck was one such person. Gerry was director of the Mennonite voluntary service program I was working for at the time, and my supervisor.[13]

I'm the kind of guy who is always trying to make sense of my life. Why was I still involved with voluntary service? What larger purpose did it serve? I believed the program was unique in the small-group dynamics it created—both among the young adult volunteers who made up the units and among the kids who came to Friendship Flat for activities.

But I began to think the model had even greater potential as an educational experience. Many of the young adults who came to D.C. as volunteers wanted to *serve*. How much more could they have gained had they also come to *learn*—had they come with the lenses of students? "Servants" focus on what they can give to others. This is a worthy endeavor but also has hints of colonialism and, being mostly whites in entirely black communities, even racism. Students, I believed, would be more ready to receive from the city, to observe, to learn.

I was a college student in the '60s. When Betty and I moved to the city, the nation was in turmoil over Dr. Martin Luther King's assassination and Vietnam, and young people were questioning everything traditional. We critiqued formal education and talked about alternatives. In the traditional classroom model, we said, pupils were spoon-fed information by lecturing teachers, and then they regurgitated what they heard in essays and exams. In contrast, real students should be able to think for themselves, to learn from experience and observation and then integrate their learning into their life work.

I began to imagine a different style of education. I wanted to bring college students to Washington for a one-year experience. They would live together in a group house and work at internships. They would take some courses at a local university to fulfill their requirements, and learn through group discussion, observation, and participation in urban life, enhanced by integrated reading and writing assignments. This would be *experiential education*, bringing students to the city to learn about how institutions function—from small nonprofits to big government—and providing college credit for the experience.

_The Players__

The idea began to gel in 1975, when the Mennonite Church decided to close the remaining voluntary service unit on South Dakota Avenue in northeast Washington. They were ready to put the large stucco house on the market.[14]

And this is where Gerry Meck became important. In fall 1975, we were at a staff retreat in Tennessee. On the ride back, Gerry and I sat, slumped in the back seat of the van, talking about changes in the voluntary service program in Washington and about the house on South Dakota Avenue. I began telling him about the little idea that was stirring around in my head.

"Well," he asked me, "if you had your druthers, what would you do?" I told him I wanted to take the voluntary service model and re-construct it so that it was viable for college students.

"If you write up a proposal," he said, "I'll go with you to present it to folks at Eastern Mennonite College."

I was in. I wrote up a very brief, unsophisticated proposal—I think it totaled two pages—and that winter, Gerry and I headed to EMC, my alma mater, to see what could be made of the thing.

On our first trip to EMC, we spoke with a few professors, the academic dean, and several students. We generated some support, but overall, EMC was not jumping on board. The institution was having cash-flow problems and looking to expand in big ways, not to start tiny, unusual programs. What's more, the deanship was in crisis, and the school's president, Myron Augsburger, who played a very public role in the wider Mennonite community, was hard to catch on campus.

I was dubious, but Gerry and I kept at it. Even though my job was ending with the closing of the second voluntary service unit, Gerry Meck agreed to keep me on his payroll while starting the new program. And they did not put the stucco house on South Dakota Avenue up for sale right away. Keeping the house meant keeping the idea alive.

Meanwhile, on EMC's campus, a young man who had met with us during our first visit to the school was catching the vision of the program. Phil Shenk started talking about spending his next year of college in the city of Washington, D.C., and, in his excitement, recruited a number of other students, too.

A history professor named Al Keim also bought into the idea. Al had been one of my professors at EMC. I remember having lunch with him when he came to D.C. with an EMC field trip that spring of 1976. We discussed the difficult situation at the college and the efforts he had made to advocate for my idea among the administration.

"I don't see how this can happen this year at EMC," he told me over lunch. "We are just having too many problems; we can't take on anything new like this right now."

"This can't wait," I insisted. "Next year will be too late. The house is available *now*. We have to act now or lose the chance."

It seemed we were stalled. The program I envisioned needed a school to endorse it by giving college credit to the students who participated. Without EMC's endorsement, I wasn't sure what I would do. I considered talking to Goshen, a Mennonite college in Indiana, but I had far fewer connections there. Maybe this was not meant to be.

When Al tells the story now, he gives credit to Chester Wenger, my father-in-law, for finally moving the proposal forward. Chester was vice-chairman of the EMC board of trustees and, apparently, concerned about his son-in-law's floundering efforts. I was married to his oldest daughter, after all.

Chester's support at the board level caused others to pay attention to this young guy in Washington—me. Somehow, thanks to Gerry, Al, Phil, and Chester, the little idea was formalized in April or May 1976. We would open our doors in late summer, and, because of Phil's recruiting efforts, we already had a group of students ready to apply.

It sometimes amazes me how this all came to be. Clearly, the birth of WSSY was a creative process. I was a networker.

The program came about because of relationships and conversations with people, not because of eloquent documents.

__Getting Started__

We were in business. It was time to put some meat on my skeleton-vision for the program. The program would have four main components: Students would live together in a group house; work at internships throughout the city; take classes at a local university (which at that time was the University of Maryland); and participate in a weekly seminar taught by WSSY staff. James Bomberger, EMC's registrar, drafted a document that explained the nuts and bolts of how this would work—how students would receive credit toward graduation for classes and work experience during their year in D.C.

I would be the program's coordinator, but I believed the job required more than my half-time position. A Goshen graduate named Arden Shank agreed to join me as a half-time assistant coordinator.

I advocated for an assistant not only because I was already juggling another half-time position[15] but also because I believed having two staff members would improve the quality of the program. I anticipated that having two leaders would provide students with greater resources when they needed support. WSSY was a holistic program—requiring a lot from students in their classes, internships, and group life. It could be emotionally demanding and stressful. Often, it seemed individual students connected to one staff person better than the other. The different personalities and gifts of each coordinator could match the needs of different students.

Having a second person involved brought in a broader range of gifts and, with the exception of Arden, gender diversity as well. I remember one time in particular that my assistant was more educated than I was. She brought a more academic focus and substance to the seminar, whereas I brought a well-developed network of organizations and internship possibilities in the city. I remain an advocate for dual or team leadership as an organizational model.

Officially, we reported directly to the dean's office. Within a year, out of the turmoil at EMC, Al Keim became dean. It was fortunate for us to have a dean who believed in our tiny, experimental program in those early years. We also pulled together an advisory board who would help oversee and support the program at a local level. The advisory board was responsible for the name that then stuck for twenty-five years. It was a good name, capturing the significant aspects of the experience: Washington Study-Service Year (WSSY), thereafter known as "Wissy."

To ease the concerns of both the college and parents, I managed to convince Miriam Weaver, a faculty member on sabbatical, to live in the house with the first batch of students.[16] Many students were looking for ways to break out of the confines of an on-campus education, and we easily enrolled nine for the first year. Phil Shenk, of course, was among them. In August 1976, the group moved in.

__Students on Board__

The next eleven years, while I served as WSSY's coordinator, were among the most rewarding in my life. I was far from perfect as a "professor," but I think my strength was in the one-on-one relationships I built with the students, as they wrestled with difficult issues in their personal lives and larger society.

I often used work-related tasks—like repairing a leaky faucet at the house or accompanying students to their internships—as opportunities for connection and conversation. I made a practice of spending one evening a week at the house—often Wednesday evening, after seminar. Usually, I joined the students for supper and then took care of needed house repairs (after helping with the dishes). This gave students an opportunity to stop by wherever I was working and talk to me.

I remember replacing a light fixture in one student's room when she happened to come by. She asked me a few questions, and what began as a friendly interaction turned into an hour-and-a-half discussion about issues she was dealing with in her personal life. I enjoyed listening to students and providing informal counseling support.

Sitting around the supper table with students was often an important time for getting feedback on the program and a window into their lives outside the seminar setting. One evening, I remember one guy slicing up watermelon for everyone and acting like a real clown. All of us were just cracking up. It was good to see students in their home setting, letting their hair down, having fun together.

♣

WSSY's early years were a lively time in the nation and the world. Students attended marches and rallies in the city. At their internships and on the streets of D.C.—and even in the classes they took at the University of Maryland—many students encountered diverse lifestyles and urban injustice in ways that challenged their more traditional upbringings.

I hoped students' WSSY experience could be relevant to their lives in the larger world. The weekly seminar was both the core of this process and the most difficult part of the program to pull off successfully. I hoped that seminar discussions could be a place for young people to explore alternatives both to the traditions they were outgrowing and the radicalism of our times.

We chose to focus seminar discussion around the institutional life of society. I was personally hesitant about the radical approach to social change that called for destroying what is, tearing down institutions, and creating new ones. We read the writings of Robert Greenleaf, who had captured my imagination during my early years in the city. Greenleaf wrote about "servant leaders" and "servant institutions." He accepted institutions as a necessary part of society. Instead of throwing them out altogether, he discussed how institutions could be made better—more humane—through responsible leadership and strong board structures.

In some senses, WSSY is one example of this middle ground I advocated. In creating the program, we questioned the limits of traditional higher education, but instead of tossing the whole thing, we created an alternative model that existed within the larger institution of EMC.

I retired from my role as WSSY coordinator in 1987. The position had given me great challenges, great joy and the opportunity to develop in three different areas: I was an administrator, a teacher, and, less officially, a counselor for students. In leaving, I was aware that I would probably never again have the opportunity to be a teacher or counselor in the way I was at WSSY, and I was sad to leave those roles behind.

__*Changes in the Years Since*__

Over the years, WSSY has evolved to accommodate the changing needs of students. It first shortened from twelve months to ten and then to nine. Today, students can choose to participate for one semester or two, allowing more flexibility for those who are on demanding academic tracks.

If you ask many of the WSSY students from the early years, they will convince you that something significant is lost in shortening the length of the experience. Many of them hold on to WSSY as a deeply formative experience in their lives. In a semester, they say, students can only get their feet wet, while the full-year program allowed for significantly more engagement with their internships and with the city at large. But as a member of the advisory board that made the decision to change, I understand that programs like WSSY must adapt to survive institutionally. I believe the one-or-two semester model is a workable compromise.

The program has changed in other ways, too. It is now called the Washington Community Scholars' Center (WCSC). The program has become much more costly as tuition prices have increased at the city universities where students take classes. And at the beginning of 2006, the program will change locations, moving from the old, stucco house on South Dakota Avenue to a newly renovated house on Taylor Street.[17]

The students have changed as well. As the 1970s became the 1980s, the excitement about social change was fading in the country. Students weren't as interested in discussing ideas and learning for learning's sake; they were more career-driven. Instead of coming to the city for urban exposure, they started coming for professional development. I suspect this shift in focus among students was partly due to the rise in tuition and, therefore, the increasing pressure to pay off debts after graduation. It was important to be employable, and their internships became their focus as a means to that end.

At its heart, though, WCSC still carries much of the original WSSY vision. It pulls students out of the limited, classroom setting—to be involved in the work world. It remains an experiment in experiential education, much as it did in 1976, integrating book-learning with urban life, seminar discussion, group living, and internships. And it continues to be formative in the lives of many young adults as they find their way and work out their identities in a changing and sometimes terrifying world.

february 19, 2005

Dad has been home from the hospital now for a week and a half. I remember the morning he woke up for the first in his very own bed. He called out to Mom, who was already up and out in the kitchen.

"Betty!" She rushed in, thinking he needed something. "The sun is shining!" he greeted her.

Since then, some days have been good, some have been hard, and all have been unpredictable. About a week ago, a blocked catheter had us rushing to an after-hours care center at two o'clock in the morning.

Before Dad came home from Washington Hospital Center, we had a railing installed out front and moved my parents' bedroom—two dressers, nightstands, and their double bed—to the first floor. Even in the face of illness and death, it is still the mundane details of life that busy our days. We wash dishes, do laundry, run to the grocery store.

We also monitor Dad's fevers, take him to the hospital for daily radiation appointments, and remember the more than thirteen medications he must take at different intervals throughout the day (with food or not, "TID" or "BID," regularly or "PRN," at bedtime or in the morning).

Ryan and Hannah have returned to Elkhart, Indiana, for now. Jason, who returned to Harrisonburg, is back this weekend, and I am glad for a companion. We brave the cold alley with a basketball and play cards every night before bed.

This morning, a small group of friends and family gathered around our living room for a service of anointing. Mom's brother, Mark, led the ritual, dipping his finger in oil and touching it delicately to Dad's forehead, over and over in the shape of a cross:

"Nelson dear, I anoint you with oil in the name of Jesus Christ for the increase of your faith and hope for the future . . . for a deeper experience of God's love addressing any regrets this turn of cancer diagnosis has brought to the surface . . . for the healing and strengthening of your body, that the cancer will recede and you will be restored to health."

Anointment of the sick is an age-old ritual that was commonly practiced among the Hebrews, and by various religious groups since. Dad remembers anointing services in the traditional Mennonite community of his childhood, where the very sick requested that a church leader (who was sometimes the farmer down the road) touch them with oil and prayer, in keeping with James 5:14.[18]

This morning's ritual and service were not about miracles but about cultivating an openness to all that is beyond our control. Dad had jotted some notes on a slip of paper from which he shared with the intimate circle in our living room. Afterward, he and I wrote down his words, as best we could remember them:

I want to express my deep thanks to each of you for interrupting your Saturday to participate in this time of special prayer for me.

This morning has somehow to do with giving myself over to the journey that has been given me; to a search for wholeness; to an openness to healing in my body and spirit.

This journey is uncharted, and I feel lost. I come to you this morning with a realization that I am broken in body and spirit, and that I need God's touch and grace—and that I need you, too, as my faith community, surrounding me.

I am, perhaps for the first time in my life, on the other side of wellness. It is a journey of great uncertainty, a journey of simply struggling to survive treatment and facing the realities of my situation, while somehow claiming hope.

This service of anointing marks for me a letting go, while reaching out for a hope in God's assurance of peace, love, and healing.

What is asked of the terminally ill seems almost impossible. On the one hand, Dad is supposed to be fighting for his life, hanging on to every last strand of hope held out before him. Uncle Mark recently sent him the movie "Rocky," in which an unknown, small-time boxer is matched against the Heavyweight Champion of the World. Mark hopes the movie will inspire in Dad a fighting spirit. Dad must not give up. He must stay optimistic. He must believe he will live.

But in the very same moment, he is preparing to die. Statistics show that half of patients with stage IV adrenocortical cancer die within the year. Very few live beyond five. We have been told that no one beats it altogether. He and Mom must revisit the language in their will and talk about finances. He must reflect on his life and think about conversations he wants to have with his children. He must prepare to say goodbye.

This is the agonizing place where reality and hope meet and have a conversation. I would like to believe Dad's final word this morning, "healing," will mean a physical cure, a shrinking of tumors, and a long and health-filled life—that the morning's oil and prayer will change the course of this disease. But I'm realizing that I am not built of optimism. And on my most cynical days, I imagine that hopefulness is a pregnant woman who carries denial in her womb.

Mom (who detests cynicism) tries to tell me that hopefulness is bigger than that. That it is possible to live in dreadful circumstances and stay, at the same time, steeped in hope. That "healing" can mean, at the very least, a deepening wellness in Dad's spirit, a readiness for whatever is to come, and that even if we do not slay Goliath like tiny, underdog David, God is with us and death does not have the final word.

These are not easy questions—nor answers.

Dad will probably die—and soon. I must hold that in one hand, because it is true. The challenge is to hold in my other hand the possibilities that lie within and beyond the probabilities. Dad says these words again and again: possibility versus probability.

I think he is finding new definitions for hope.

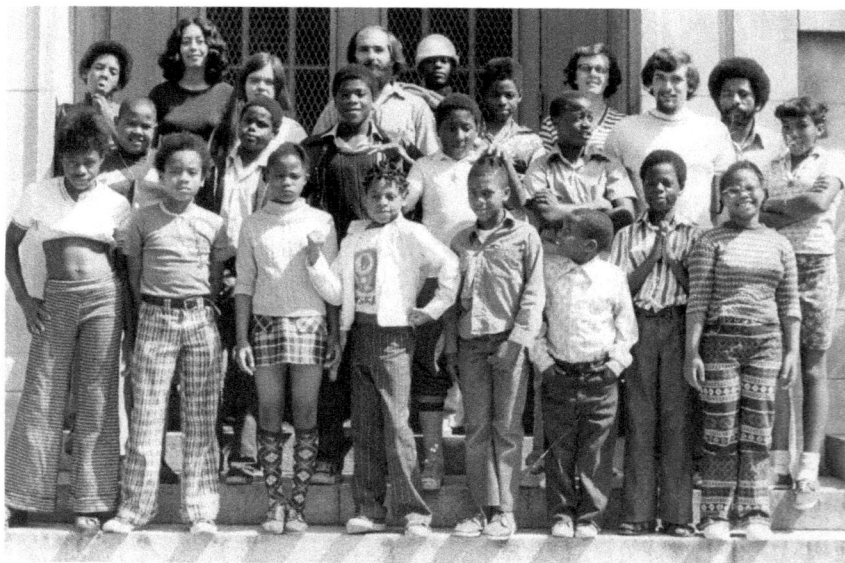

Learning Center students and staff strike a pose for the camera, circa 1975. Photo submitted by Herb and Ginny Buckwalter

Chapter 3

THE LEARNING CENTER

Daughter's Voice
Imperfection

I was surprised to learn one year at Christmas that Dad had listened to Johnny Cash when he was younger. When I was a child, we had very little popular music in our home—I would never have guessed Dad was familiar with Johnny Cash at all. But there it was on his "wish list," the clues our family passes around at Christmastime so we can give each other better gifts. Pretty soon, a Johnny Cash Golden Hits album made its way under the tree.

Well, sings Cash in "Man in Black," *you wonder why I always dress in black.* The answer? *I wear the black for the poor and the beaten down, livin' in the hopeless, hungry side of town.*

Dad rarely talked theology (nor did he dress in black) but underneath his serious commitments and work in D.C. was the New Testament's Sermon on the Mount, in which Jesus turns normal thinking on its head with crazy-talk. You just struck a million-dollar deal and think you've got it made? Think again. For "woe to you who are rich," he says in Luke. And woe to you as well if you are well-fed and laughing and praised by all your friends.

But blessed are the poor, the hungry, and all of you who are walking through valleys of depression and loss, he says. Blessed are the despised among you, the feared, forgotten, ghettoized.

Oh, and by the way, "love your enemies, do good, and lend, expecting nothing in return."[19]

Like many others before and since—and possibly like Cash himself—Dad believed that all of us are endowed with a God-given responsibility: to name the world's injustices and to work patiently and relentlessly to change, tweak, or completely upset the systems that create them.

My parents and their Mennonite friends were not the only church-raised folks thinking outside the box at their small-group gatherings and meetings. Through the 1960s and 1970s, a number of faith-based-activist-types in the city were finding one another and forming churches and communities. These creative and idealistic groups composed the social and spiritual geography in which my parents planted themselves. It proved to be fertile soil for a number of my dad's involvements.

One of these groups was the ecumenical Church of the Saviour, founded in the 1940s by Gordon and Mary Cosby.[20] While many churches and denominations are built on shared *beliefs*, the Church of the Saviour was built instead on shared *practices*, and was very active in social causes. Members of the church gathered for worship on Sunday mornings. Through the rest of the week, they met in smaller "mission groups," which, over the years, were responsible for developing a number of nonprofit organizations in the city.

In 1965, a group from the Church of the Saviour founded For Love of Children (FLOC), an organization working to serve troubled families and foster children.[21] Six years later, FLOC provided the organizational umbrella under which my parents and a number of their friends would start a school called the Learning Center.

The FLOC Learning Center was begun as an alternative day school for foster children with special needs. These were

children who were failing out of the public school system—
kids who were generally falling through the cracks. During the
school's early and shaky years, a small team of volunteer teachers struggled to control the students' sometimes outrageous behavior.

Dad became the Learning Center's half-time administrator
in 1973, its third year, having no idea he would stay on for the
next thirteen. In 2005, greatly weakened by cancer, Dad reflected on his years with the school. "When I look back now,"
he told me, "it's amazing I did not burn out."

♣

In Dad's life, his Christian faith was the background music,
while his sociological analyses and day-to-day work in the
world were the featured performance. And, as I've said before,
his strongest act was his staying power, an enormous capacity to
stick with efforts that seemed tipped toward failure from the
outset.

Even when he knew they were imperfect, he did not let the
projects' deficiencies immobilize him. He worked toward more
just and healthy structures, operating on the faith that even
flawed projects are sometimes better than their alternatives. As
my dad spoke about the Learning Center, for example, I heard
in his words a determination to improve on the weaknesses he
had identified at Friendship Flat.

This is a good lesson for critics like me and many of my
generation who prefer to see the flaws in others' efforts without
ever initiating our own. Many of us assume we must first develop an area of expertise before we are qualified to act, so we sit
back, read books, criticize, go to graduate school, and wait on
the experts. Maybe we don't try because what we most fear is
our own failure.

As Dad describes it, Vivian Headings was one of the group
that was largely responsible for the Learning Center's birth.
They—like so many of my parents' friends—were willing to

envision something they knew very little about. It didn't matter that Vivian had not written a dissertation on educating troubled kids. It did not matter that she was a nurse, not a teacher. What mattered was that she and the others saw desperation in the city's system of warehousing children and felt called to address it.[22]

Recently, Vivian and I were laughing about this very thing—how the Learning Center was begun by a group of people who, for the most part, had little idea what they were doing. "You know, looking back on all that," she said, "I do believe it is possible for committed groups of people to envision changes and make things happen."

Vivian's words are inspiring. It's the stuff of survival stories and graduation speeches, right? *Dream. Believe. Things will unfold that you never imagined, and you will be part of making them happen.* But to me, this is only the beginning of a long and unresolved conversation about what good social-change work really looks like.

Many of us have heard at least one story of a well-meaning group who started up a project in some down-and-out neighborhood in such-and-such a city or faraway country—only to pack out early, leaving in their wake more harm than change for the better. Often, these groups are following a vision without proper training, research, and analysis of their given contexts.

A friend of mine has been working with nurses, doctors, and community organizers hoping to provide Spanish-speaking health services to immigrants in South Philadelphia. She tells me that their efforts were initially met with some resistance from neighbors who have seen several groups pass through in the past, asking residents to fill out surveys and participate in discussions. These groups claimed that they would address the community's needs with a new health clinic or education center, but nothing sustainable ever came of their good intentions. The mostly Latino residents were left feeling used and distrustful.[23]

The story of the Learning Center is *not* such a story, but could it have been? What makes it different? Not much, I think, especially in the early years. According to Dad's telling of the story, the whole project nearly collapsed on more than one occasion. So what are the reasons the Learning Center lasted and did so much good for hurting children, when other similar efforts have failed? I credit that staying power I keep talking about and the help of a few folks with more experience and expertise; plus a little faith, good luck, and—eventually—the transfer of leadership into African-American hands.

Fred Taylor, who served as FLOC's executive director from 1966 through 2002, met me for lunch several months after Dad's death. He remembers the words of a sociologist who did some consulting for the Learning Center in its early years. *If the Learning Center had only a benign effect on its students,* she claimed, *even if the children gained nothing from it, they would still be better off than they would be in the public school system.* The public schools at that time were so ill-equipped in responding to students with emotional, behavioral, and learning difficulties that they regularly sent the children home at lunchtime.

Fred went on to describe for me the only time he remembers seeing my dad cry. The two of them were meeting to discuss the Learning Center, which was having significant trouble managing behavior in the program's early years. Dad was feeling helpless in the face of the school's problems and the staff's limited experience, including his own. His stress—and worry that the school would not make it through—was spilling out in sighs and tears.

"I don't know either what we're going to do about this," Fred remembers telling Dad, "but tomorrow is another day."

With the help of some new and experienced staff, the Learning Center did survive its most unstable years. It was approved by the city as a special education school, and by the time it closed in 2005, the Learning Center enrolled about forty students a year and employed a capable, largely African-American teaching staff.

♣

Six months after Dad died, Dan Charles, a writer and family friend, agreed to read an earlier version of this book's manuscript. By the second chapter, he was already circling a word that appeared again and again in my Dad's vernacular: *model, model, model*. No, he was not talking about Kate Moss and Geena Davis. In the face of the world's injustice, Johnny Cash wrote songs, others wrote letters, marched, and spent time in prison. Dad? He preferred to look at the structure of organizations and programs, discuss improvements, implement them. He preferred to talk about models.

Of Friendship Flat, he says: "over-dependency remained a problem inherent to the voluntary service *model*." In WSSY, he wanted to "take the voluntary service *model* and re-construct it so that it was viable for college students." Of the Learning Center, he comments: "Relying on completely unpaid staff was an unsustainable *model*."

Dan and I debated, editorially, what to do with the over-abundance of the word. In the end, we agreed: Model was one of Dad's favorite words, central to the way the world looked through his eyes, essential to how he interpreted it. The word, as much as possible, had to stay. I did replace it in some instances with near-synonyms like "structure," "organization," and "example," but I chose to leave it as "model" everywhere else.

It's as though social change was a slow-moving train, and while others focused on its shiny color or its destination, Dad obsessed with the machinery behind the paint, the joints that needed oil, the fact that the railroad's employee configuration needed restructuring.

This concern with structure and model makes Dad's explanation of things tedious at times. Most of us would rather get on the train and go somewhere than talk about how it works. Yet I am not sure that any of the imperfect efforts Dad describes in this book would have survived were it not for his interest in their machinery.

Father's Voice
For Love of Children

L ooking back, I can hardly believe what we did. We were a group of young adults who wanted to bring lasting change to the children in Washington's child welfare system. So we pooled our gifts and called on others for additional support and training. In 1971, under the umbrella of a larger organization called For Love of Children (FLOC), we opened an alternative day school for foster children and others with special education needs. Initially, I became involved in small ways, drawn by our group's shared concern for children so neglected by D.C.'s social systems. Eventually, though, I developed a far closer relationship to the FLOC Learning Center than I could have imagined.

__*The Problem with Junior Village*__

Not long after Betty and I arrived in Washington, a friend introduced me to a man named Fred Taylor. Fred was a serious man, tall with a slender frame and gentle manner. His friendship and influence on my life continue to this day.

Fred was involved in developing For Love of Children, an organization concerned with the city's neglect of disadvantaged children. Through public advocacy and social services, FLOC sought an alternative approach to serving broken families.

During the fall of 1968, our first year at Friendship Flat, Betty and I and our four fellow volunteers took a class Fred was offering on the city's inadequate services to children and families. In short, the "white flight" of the '60s had left inner-city

Washington deficient of taxes and services, while the influx of low-income families—many of them African-Americans moving into the city from the South—created more need. In this context, unemployment, evictions, and homelessness were common.

Police were finding children unattended or in at-risk situations. Their answer was to take children from their parents and put them in a large custodial institution in lower southeast called Junior Village. Its critics called it a "warehouse for children and youth." Junior Village was made up of cottages that together held up to 900 kids and was extremely overcrowded.[24]

In Fred's 1968 class, he encouraged those of us in the room toward greater consciousness of our social context. How could we—and society as a whole—better meet the needs of children and families? From my point of view, it helped our whole voluntary service unit become more than simply "good helpers." We became more sophisticated in our understandings of children and family needs, and more aware of how our approach could foster either greater empowerment or dependency in the children who came to Friendship Flat.

The seeds of my interest in children and family concerns—and then for my involvement in developing the FLOC Learning Center—really lay in my experiences as a volunteer on W Street. Friendship Flat had mostly floundered in its efforts to bring lasting changes to the community. In helping to open the FLOC Learning Center a few years later, I hoped to develop an institution that, while still imperfect, would better model the change I envisioned for society.

♣

Fred's class cultivated a real connection between him and me, and our relationship continued through my two years as a volunteer and beyond. Fred had a particular interest in developing a connection to Mennonites because he knew that there were Mennonites volunteering at Junior Village.

Mennonite Central Committee (MCC) placed volunteers at Junior Village in hopes that they could be a "healing presence" to children in need. The MCCers were clearly terrific people, and the children loved them. But Fred explained to me that he saw their efforts differently. Their compassionate presence, he believed, was actually enabling a bad institution to continue. He wanted MCC to "jump tracks"—to join FLOC in calling for institutional change. Just as I had discovered at Friendship Flat, caring relationships certainly brought positive change at a personal level for individual children, but lasting change would have to be structural.

__The Beginnings of an Idea__

After Betty and I moved from Friendship Flat to our first apartment, we gathered with about ten other friends on Sunday evenings, sometimes for discussion and sometimes just for fellowship.[25] All of us were from Mennonite backgrounds, and some of us were aware of Fred's concerns about MCC and Junior Village. In January 1971, *The Washington Post* started running articles about the less-than-adequate conditions at Junior Village, revealing the underbelly of the city's warehouse for neglected children.

These articles were creating quite a stir in the city and became part of our discussion one Sunday evening when the person in our group who was to lead our gathering did not show up. Vivian Headings, one of our group, was already involved in FLOC's work, and these issues were close to her heart. She told us that she felt called to create an alternative to Junior Village and to challenge MCC to a different means of addressing the situation. She wondered if our group, as Mennonites, could play a unique role. Would anyone else join her, she asked, in exploring ways of responding to the plight of D.C.'s children?[26]

At the outset, a small group, including Betty, came forward. They met at Verle and Vivian's house and began developing a vision for a group foster home that would be open

specifically to children who were failing in school—children
with special educational needs. One-on-one support at the
home would help these children stay in school. It would be
staffed with volunteers, including, the group hoped, MCCers.
Instead of simply propping up a failing institution like Junior
Village, the home would model an alternative and give MCC a
different way of investing its energy.

We asked Fred Taylor to come to our Sunday evening gathering when the group presented this idea. He listened carefully
and was very affirming of the group's thinking. He then responded with a different suggestion.

"I want to encourage you to consider something else," he
said. "Instead of starting a foster home, what about a day
school?" A small school, he reasoned, could help children from
various foster homes and difficult situations get back on track.
This could actually benefit more children in more families. He
also shared his observation that the massive problems FLOC
children were having in the public school system were actually
threatening the future and stability of some of the foster homes.

Fred's question nudged the group in a new direction. *What
about a day school?* At this point, I started getting involved, too.
We, of course, knew almost nothing about what it would take
to start a school, but we had a vision and a considerable amount
of collective experience. We began working to make it happen.

♣

Some time earlier, a man named Gilbert Johnson had visited Lancaster County and befriended an Amish farmer. He
was deeply impressed with the Amish way of life, especially
their emphasis on peace and service to others. When Gil left
Lancaster, the farmer suggested that he look for a Mennonite
church where he lived, explaining that Mennonites and Amish
shared similar beliefs and values. This is how Gilbert Johnson
discovered Hyattsville Mennonite Church just a few blocks
from his home and soon became involved in the congregation.

We learned of Gilbert Johnson because two of the couples in our Sunday-evening group also attended Hyattsville Mennonite Church. As it turned out, he became key in developing the plan for the Learning Center. He was an experienced educator, and trained teachers for a living. He had a much better sense than the rest of us what ingredients were necessary for making a school workable, not to mention acceptable to the public officials who would eventually approve it as a special education school.

The group of us developed a proposal and took it to the FLOC governing council. We outlined our plans for the school's first year, including a (tiny) ten-thousand-dollar budget, which we raised pretty much internally. The council approved the proposal. Bob Wert found a church—Sixth Presbyterian—willing to rent us their basement. And, to make a longer story short, the FLOC Learning Center opened its doors around Thanksgiving 1971.

__*The First Years*__

During its first year, the school had nine students, mostly from FLOC foster homes. The number increased to twelve by the end of the school year. My primary contribution at the beginning was in recruiting a staff of volunteer teachers. Through my voluntary service connections, friends, and family, I recruited five teachers, each with unique housing arrangements according to their situations and needs.[27] From that point on, I gradually became more involved in birthing and running the school.

The five teachers worked together as a team, with no principal. Gil Johnson would often stop by the school during the day to help the teachers develop methods of dealing with behavioral problems. Relying on a completely volunteer staff was unsustainable, but we pulled it off for the Learning Center's first two years. We used our ten-thousand-dollar budget mostly for rent and supplies.

Undergirding the staff was the "Learning Center support group," which became a significant piece of the organizational structure. The support group consisted of some of those who had originally envisioned the school, as well as a few others—like me and Gil Johnson—who had become involved in the meantime. All the teachers were welcome to attend as well. We met every other week for a potluck supper, to review how things were going at the school and to discuss any needs and concerns.

The Learning Center would not have lasted long without the support group. History provides story after story of new life and necessary change emerging from small citizen groups working together around a common concern. The Learning Center support group brought sustainability to the vision, providing support and perspective even as staff came and went.

__My Years as Administrator__

In 1973, a number of changes in my life made my time more flexible. I was finishing graduate school at Catholic University, with a Master's degree in Sociology. Betty had finished a year earlier and now had a steady job as a family and marriage counselor. I was still overseeing the two Mennonite voluntary service units, but Friendship Flat was closing. I had also been working as a Red Top cab driver in Arlington, but one of my passengers had recently held me up at gunpoint, and soon afterward I decided I would not drive cab again.

At about the same time, the Learning Center, now two years old, was in need of more administrative oversight. Sixth Presbyterian Church was tired of our using their basement, and some of our volunteer staff had plans to leave the city at the end of their two-year service assignments. The support group was feeling overwhelmed.

In March 1973, I agreed to help find a new space and address funding and staffing concerns—for a minimal salary. As it turned out, I would work half-time as the Learning Center's administrator for the next thirteen years, becoming involved in a much more expansive way than I expected. In a sense, I took on the role of an executive director. I made financial decisions and was the ongoing link to FLOC, Fred Taylor, and the FLOC Board, who officially had authority over the Learning Center. I was also the ongoing link to the Learning Center support group who, unofficially, provided much of the oversight, while the FLOC Board was overloaded by other programs. When I look back now, it's amazing I did not burn out.

During my first year as half-time administrator, aspects of the Learning Center had become extremely chaotic. One of my first challenges was finding a new location for the school. I negotiated a new space in a former high school building that was sitting empty across from where Betty and I lived. The Learning Center moved into the new building for that third year and took on new students.

The make-up of our staff brought more challenges. Key teachers left and new ones came on. The Learning Center was not insulated from the complexities of racism that surrounded us. We were very aware at the school's beginning that we were dependent on mostly white-controlled resources, and our volunteer staff were mostly white. But we knew an African-American presence was essential, as all our students were black. We did not want to perpetuate stereotypes by having our students associate their betterment with whiteness.

It was difficult to hire African-American teachers from the local community because we did not, at first, have the financial resources to compete with the other opportunities available to black professionals in the city. With time—and more money—the Learning Center developed a black identity. The leadership and teaching staff were eventually predominantly African-American.

In our third year, we started paying the teachers modest salaries, so we wouldn't be as dependent on volunteers. We also succeeded in getting the program approved by the city as a special education school. The city gave $2,300 per approved child. Getting approved brought us greater credibility and a stronger financial base, but it also had a downside. The city now classified us strictly as a special education program. This labeled our students and limited the kinds of children we could serve. Rather than taking students who were just showing signs of failure, we could now accept only children who were already failing badly.

Before long, the city was referring us kids with more difficulties, serious learning disabilities, and clinical diagnoses. The Learning Center began providing a greater number of specialized services to help meet the children's needs, bringing in reading specialists, counselors, and family social workers from outside the school.

♣

As the school's administrator, I didn't have much direct contact with students. This distance from the emotional intensity of the school may explain, in part, how I managed to stay so long in such a highly stressful situation. There were a few times I became more involved. I remember one boy in particular whose behavior was hard to manage during my first year. He was probably about twelve years old and, as with most of the children in the school, would likely have been a normal kid if it weren't for his stressful and impoverished home situation.

Our teachers had run out of ideas for how to manage his behavior, and one day he became so out of control and dangerous we asked him to go home in the middle of the day. He of course refused. If he wouldn't go himself, we would take him. I remember driving the whole way across the city while one of our teachers physically restrained the boy in the back seat of the car. I worried what would happen if someone stopped us and called the police. Situations like this were deeply unsettling to all of us whose principal ideal was compassion, whose principal hope was to create a better life for these kids.

During my first year as the school's administrator, we had more behavioral problems than we were equipped to manage. It was so tough one of our new teachers would scream in his car on his way to work—scream therapy, it was called—to help reduce his anxiety. I remember feeling like it was getting out of hand and worrying that we might have to close the school.

I was so overwhelmed. I would sometimes think to myself, *If this fails, I can always go back to the farm.* Knowing I had a fallback option was somehow comforting and allowed me to pour myself into my work with the Learning Center.

The school was desperate for help in managing behavior. Then, onto the scene came Chris Donaldson.[28] Chris had been a teacher in a number of settings, working with emotionally disturbed kids. When he applied to the Learning Center in the middle of my first year, I was aware that Chris had a history of mental illness, which was part of the reason we were able to recruit him—he was having a hard time finding a job elsewhere. I was somewhat torn but ultimately decided to take the risk of hiring him because he had so much experience and confidence in working with students like ours.

To tell you the truth, I am not sure we could have done it without Chris. He really turned the school around. He had a gift in relating to difficult kids and helped the team of teachers finally institute an effective behavioral management system. Teachers kept track of students' good behavior with points on the blackboard. Twice a day, the children were rewarded based on the number of points they had earned. At the end of the week, those who had accumulated enough points got a special prize—like a field trip to the zoo. The technique worked because it consistently reinforced positive behavior.

Chris brought a tighter structure to the Learning Center, replacing what had been a more flexible, creative, and open approach. The school's overarching goal, of course, was to teach reading, writing, and arithmetic, but too many behavioral problems were making this almost impossible. With Chris's technique, teachers and kids had very clear expectations of what was to happen each day. It kept teachers busy keeping track of points on the board—but, most importantly, it also kept the school under control so teaching could happen.

With the help of Chris Donaldson and, later, a child psychologist who came regularly to work with our staff, the Learning Center's teachers got better and better. Our students were mostly between eight and fifteen years old, referred by the foster care system or the city's special education department. We processed their applications and, if accepted, divided them by age into three to four classrooms. They often brought more than learning disabilities to school. Some brought histories of physical abuse, homelessness, and parents struggling with addiction. All came from impoverished backgrounds.

♣

Over the summer, I had Chris doing some work at the FLOC offices. He began doing slightly wacky things. When he left the room, he expected other employees—who were working for completely different programs—to answer his phone. He acted like he was the chief executive of the place. It was clear he was losing some touch with reality.

As the teachers came back to the Learning Center for the fall semester, Chris' behavior got stranger. He would sometimes show up in the mornings with his eyes glazed over, telling funny and unrealistic stories. Things he would say created misunderstandings among the staff, and other teachers were uncomfortable around him. Some of his behaviors seemed potentially violent.

It was hard for me to accept that the same guy who had come in about eight months before and saved our school was now, himself, a problem. I confronted Chris and told him he would have to shape up to keep his job. To my great relief, he cooperated. With some time off and resumed medications, he improved significantly. That next year was one of our best.

It was the following year, however, that things really fell apart for Chris. Classes had been in session for several weeks when a mother claimed that he had hit her son, who was a student at the school. Chris denied it. I found myself in a difficult position. Should I believe the mother, or stand by my teacher? What if he then abused other kids and put the whole school in jeopardy?

I decided to support Chris but promised that we would monitor his behavior more closely. There were no more reports of physical abuse toward kids, but there were signs again of a mental health breakdown. Soon afterward, his wife left him. His mental stability crumbled quickly. And so, after watching this man salvage the Learning Center when the rest of us were at our wit's end, I finally had to let Chris Donaldson go. The school would have to continue without him.

__Another Imperfect Project__

With all the chaos of the Learning Center's early years, I had good reason to become cynical. Here I was once again amid what seemed to be a flawed enterprise. I understood, however, that projects go through phases. At this early and very uncertain stage, I acted on the faith that better phases were to come. It would take patience to see the fruition of our efforts.

I accepted, too, that of all models for social change and community betterment, none is pure. All are flawed. I did believe the design of some projects to be better than others, and the Learning Center was, at the very least, considerably more humane and effective than Junior Village.

With its connections to the public school and foster care systems, I wondered if the Learning Center also had a better chance of creating institutional change than did Friendship Flat. Overall, I think this proved true. The Learning Center was easier to explain to the community. It was approved by the city as a day school that served special-needs kids, giving it an acceptable and understandable legitimacy. We also discovered, however, that becoming more institutionalized and legitimate in the eyes of the community limited our flexibility and creativity.

Hiring a competent and professional African-American staff and bringing in specialized services were positive and necessary changes but also significantly more costly. We constantly needed money, so fundraising and financial management became key parts of my job.

Increasingly, the school's staff had less and less connection with the informal Learning Center support group, though it remained an important support for me, personally, in my work with the school. The fact that the support group continued to be mostly white was a noticeable weakness in the organization's structure. Eventually, the Learning Center staff took on many of the support group's responsibilities, solving problems and envisioning future direction at weekly staff conferences, and the support group faded out.

♣

I was the Learning Center's half-time administrator until December 1986, six months before I also retired from the Washington Study-Service Year program.[29] For five of my final years, Marlin Good worked as the school's program director, while I handled most administrative tasks. Marlin and I were cousins, and we worked well together. I had called him when he was finishing up graduate work, and the Learning Center was desperate for leadership trained in special education. Somehow, in my persistence, I convinced Marlin to move to D.C., with his very pregnant wife Barb, and take the job. I don't know if I could have done it without him. After Marlin left the school, however, I had more conflict with the program directors who followed and felt limited by my role as administrator.

The school increasingly needed a "chief cook and bottle-washer," someone who had both administrative and programmatic functions. In my leaving, roles shifted, and the program director became school principal, taking on more of the responsibilities I had carried. The position of half-time administrator was discontinued; in fact, I was the only person ever to hold that title at the Learning Center.

__*Endings*__

The Learning Center was designed as a short-term intervention for children failing out of the public school system. Junior Village so disrupted a child's life and created such dependency that it seemed impossible they would ever re-enter the mainstream. At the Learning Center, we tried to maintain as much normalcy as possible for the children. After two or three years, we hoped our students would gain enough from the Learning Center's specialized setting to re-integrate into D.C. public schools. This remained our vision, even as the seriousness of the students' needs made re-integration harder to achieve.

Today, the Learning Center is more than thirty years old. By now, the school has outlived the involvement of any of its original founders. It enrolls about forty students a year and is located in the basement of the Thurgood Marshall Center.[30] To many people's great disappointment, FLOC has run into significant financial problems and is closing a number of its programs this year. It looks like the 2004-2005 school year may be the Learning Center's last.[31]

I feel some sense of loss, of course, in that something I helped give birth to is coming to an end. But I do believe some organizations have limited life spans. It may be that the Learning Center has served its time, making positive impacts in many children's lives at a time when few services were available to them. Today, a broader variety of public charter schools and special education programs will provide failing students with options even after the Learning Center is gone.

The Learning Center was a big piece of my service to the city and was deeply rewarding. Although it was never a clear success, the Learning Center embodied for me an important ideal: Social change must happen at individual *and* institutional levels. At the Learning Center, we attempted personal change through teacher-student relationships and structural change by modeling an alternative to existing systems, pushing schools to have more concern for kids with special needs.

Society's trend is toward large-scale institutional structures, and schools are no exception. Sometimes, small schools close while bigger ones survive because they are, proportionately, less costly and because their larger size can allow for more specialized services. But larger schools are impersonal, and many kids fall through the cracks.

I believe the Learning Center did a better job than most D.C. public schools in our efforts to provide personalized attention to troubled kids. In partnership with FLOC's programs, we hoped to address the children's needs for more than simple reading, writing, and arithmetic. Much bigger, more complex problems—poverty, family breakdown, and personal violence—surround many children in U.S. cities, and I wonder if we as a society must shift away from big, so-called efficient institutions to smaller, personalized models of education—as we tried to model at the Learning Center.

march 29, 2005

I have been reading up on adrenocortical cancer (ACC). I can tell you where the adrenal glands are located in the body and that ACC is most likely to metastasize first to the lungs and liver. I can tell you that only one in two million people get the disease and that the drug most commonly used to treat it is called mitotane.

In the end, though, no one understands why some bodies respond to the drug while most don't. In the end, no one knows why the cancer kills some people and leaves others to live a few years longer. In the end, we know so very little. Our bodies remain mysterious even in the twenty-first century. My little threads of hope rest in that mystery.

Three weeks ago, Dad developed significant soreness in his right hip which brought us yet another treatment decision: If the pain was caused by tumor activity in the bone, would it be best to reduce it and prevent possible fracture through targeted radiation treatments? Radiation would postpone Dad's participation in a clinical trial at the National Institute of Health (NIH) designed specifically for ACC patients. He would probably undergo a more traditional chemotherapy regimen instead, alongside the nightly doses of mitotane.

The twists and forks and dead-ends are constant and confusing. I wish we had a map.

At NIH, scans confirmed the development of a tumor in Dad's right front pelvis. With the help of our NIH physician, Doctor Fojo, we decided that Dad would undergo traditional radiation for two weeks. After that, he would begin chemotherapy infusions of a drug called cisplatin instead of joining the NIH clinical trial.

In the world of cancer, we rely on percentages and statistics to provide a cold, rugged guide in making decisions and gauging our hopefulness. In the case of ACC in particular, statistics are sketchy at best, as the disease—and therefore clinical studies of patients—are so rare. Still we try to sift through how many of what kind of patients have responded in what way to which treatments. We have no proof that the NIH trial would have been more successful than the cisplatin chemotherapy. So far, the trial's results have not been any stronger than traditional therapies, all of which rarely work. Yet it is hard to give up the chance.

At Dad's first radiation appointment, specialists lightly tattoo his skin so their lasers will hit precisely the same spot every time. Dad describes the equipment they use in administering the radiation, otherworldly machines with metal electronic arms that rotate slowly around his body, while he lies flat and alone in the dim room. I don't know what of this is true and what I have imagined. I have never been inside.

Dad had his last appointment on Friday, and the radiation seems to have relieved the pain in his hip enough that he can walk short distances without a wheelchair. We celebrate. These days, small victories are worth celebrating.

Now we brace ourselves for the next assault: We go in tomorrow for Dad's first cisplatin infusion, in which he will lie on a hospital bed for four hours while toxins flow quietly into his veins.

Meanwhile, he has also been taking increasingly large doses of mitotane, a drug used specifically in treating ACC patients. Dad concentrates on deliberately swallowing the large, bitter pills each evening. As the drug builds up in his blood stream, his body responds queasily. Eating is becoming a challenge.

Studies vary but show that, at best, one in four patients responds to mitotane. And "response," the oncologist clarified for anyone whose hopes were creeping a little too high, does not mean "cure." In some cases, it means only that the drug slightly stunts the growth of the ever-developing tumors.

More than forty years ago, as I understand it, mitotane was an ingredient in certain insecticides. Some farm workers using the insecticides developed problems with their adrenal gland, so today, the drug is used to attack adrenal cells gone awry. Go figure.

Is cancer the only disease in which we treat sick people by making them sicker? Decades from now, we will no doubt look back incredulously at our use of toxins to heal the ill among us.

So we move into tomorrow, and the day after that, wondering which side effects will be the worst, wondering if this is all for naught, hoping with everything that it isn't.

In the past, Dad has shared aloud with me some of his thoughts and feelings but has spent much more time listening to mine. The terrors of the past two months, however, have opened him to me like a cantaloupe, his seeds and juices spilling between us, where we can slide them between our fingers and into our mouths. Depression. Gratitude. Grief. Unending love. I have never felt so close to him.

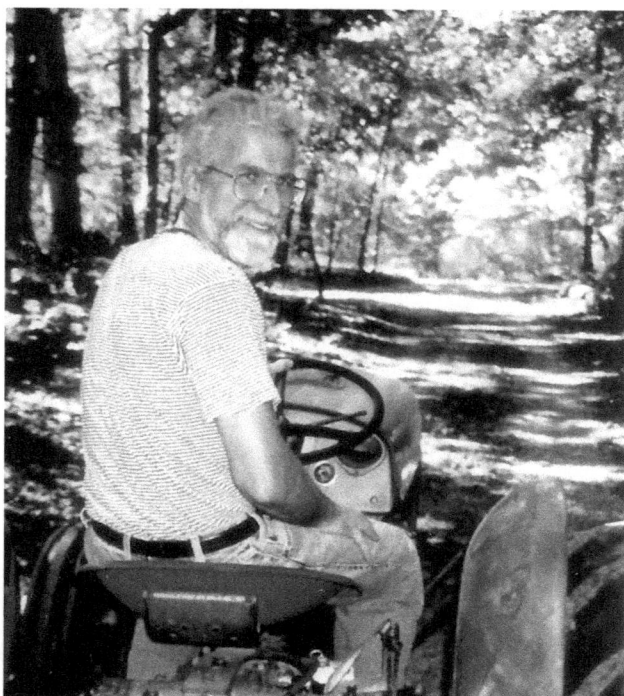

Nelson looks right at home on the seat of his childhood-farm tractor, as he pulls a wagon-full of children on a hayride. Photo credit: Cheryl Martin, Rolling Ridge, 1998

Chapter 4

ROLLING RIDGE

Daughter's Voice
Risk-No-Risk Living

I was a senior in college and leaving for a trip with six friends. We were driving in a minivan borrowed from my parents to Fort Benning, Georgia, for the annual School of the Americas protest, a four-day endeavor in all.[32] To fit all seven friends and our gear into the minivan, we each had to take very little. In short, we planned to more or less wear the same outfits several days in a row.

Dad called me before we hit the road. Even though I had left home when I was sixteen to live with my grandparents and had proven a fairly independent and responsible young woman, my dad still had a tendency to seemingly micro-manage my life: "So, what did you pack?" I rolled my eyes at the unnecessary question. Maybe it was my dad's way of showing love—caring about the details.

"Well, we had to pack light, so I have two shirts and clean underpants. But I think I'll just wear the same pair of jeans all weekend." Then came a question I didn't quite expect.

"One pair of pants? What if they *split*?" It had crossed my mind that I might be in for a rather uncomfortable weekend if it happened to rain and I was stuck in wet denim for the long trip home, but it had never occurred to me that the pants might tear, nor that this would be a problem.

"*Dad*," I groaned. "Believe me, they will not split. And if they do, I'll be at a *protest*. There will be lots of people with ripped jeans."

That was that. I headed off to Georgia with a carload of friends, snacks, and big ideas about the world . . . and one pair of jeans. I'm sure you can guess what happened next. Day three in Georgia, I stepped up onto some bleachers for a better view and, sure enough, ripped my one and only pair of pants, right in the crotch.

I hated it when Dad was right.

The point is this: Dad was one of the most thorough and careful guys I have ever met, especially when it came to his family. He planned our summer camping trips with meticulous detail and made sure to pack provisions for any kind of obstacle we might encounter on the way. The cars he and Mom owned over the years—even when old and slightly clunky—were always well-serviced and stocked with tools, rags, jumper cables, flashlights, maps, extra oil, a small broom, and, in case we were ever stuck in a snowy mess, cat litter for traction.

As I have already described, Dad kept our basketball hoop locked to prevent problems in the alley behind our house. He was known to walk young adults home after small group or church meetings in my parents' living room, to make sure they made it safely. He and Mom locked windows and doors every night and then double-checked them. He took every precaution, prepared for every misfortune.

Yet, at the same time, Dad was an enormous risk-taker. He took on more than one risky project in his life, throwing his weight behind idealistic visions with no promise that their outcomes would be worth his time and effort. He never made a lot of money, often relied on my mom's employer for health insurance, and put a long list of things ahead of job security.

In this chapter, Dad tells the story of Rolling Ridge. From its beginning, this proved to be yet another risky vision that, at certain points, had Dad diving in practically to the point of drowning. His deep commitment was not without consequences and probably put more strain on his marriage and family life than any other challenge he took on—even the cancer that finally killed him.

♣

Rolling Ridge Study Retreat Community is the name of a small intentional community and ecumenical retreat center on 1,400 wooded acres near Harpers Ferry, West Virginia. Of all Dad's involvements, this one may have been the closest to his heart. Like the Learning Center, Rolling Ridge was a vision born in living rooms and around dining room tables in the sixties and seventies. Dad was involved nearly from the outset.

By the time I was a toddler in the 1980s, my parents and three other couples had solidified into a group that would be the primary force behind developing the "study retreat community" they envisioned, and—perhaps more importantly— they had acquired land on which their vision could grow.

In 1982, our family moved to the tract of tree-covered land in West Virginia for the summer. I was not yet two years old, Ryan was four, and my younger brother, Jason, was barely a thought in my parents' minds. There was not much there in those days—a rugged house previously occupied by a mountain family, a geodesic dome covered in plastic, a cook shed, and lots of space for camping. There was also a small one-room cottage, where we would spend the next five months with no toilet and no electricity—an experience we have always referred to as our "sabbatical" from city life.

As both my brothers and I transformed from toddlers into children over the next few years, Mom lessened her involvement with the Rolling Ridge group while Dad poured ever more time and energy into the project.

In the years since, I have been to Rolling Ridge for count-less church retreats, youth work camps, and family vacations. Wonderful people have built homes on the land, planted a gar-den, and become a community. Other than our five-month sabbatical, our family never lived at Rolling Ridge. Even so, it became for me a home away from home, a refuge from the city. Dad's involvement was so longstanding and significant that many considered him an honorary member of the residential volunteer staff and community.

Down the hill and across the creek from the community's homes, the opposite hillside is spotted with retreat facilities, in-cluding a six-bedroom retreat house built largely on my dad's back. His leadership in the construction of the Retreat House at a time when forward movement was slow and frustrating was one of Dad's most significant contributions to Rolling Ridge—and the one that most nearly broke him.

The Retreat House has become meaningful for church and community groups from the D.C. area who come regularly to spend time together and enjoy a respite from the urban rush and bustle. This was the keystone of Dad's vision for what Rolling Ridge could be.

"Some urban families maintain privately owned beach homes and mountain cabins where they can go for breaks from city life," Dad told me. "My hope has been that Rolling Ridge could serve a similar purpose, allowing families to hold a con-nection to a piece of land outside the city—and to the larger natural world—without the financial burden of owning and maintaining it themselves."

This is possible through the "partner group model" which Dad describes later in this chapter. This financial arrangement not only gave Rolling Ridge some of the capital it needed to build the Retreat House but over the years has created a bridge, giving several hundred people a sense of relationship and re-sponsibility to Rolling Ridge; to its mountains, creeks, and wa-terfalls; to entire congregations of trees—and to each other.

In 2007, nearly two years after Dad's death, I moved to Rolling Ridge for the summer. I lived with Keith and Rachelle Lyndaker Schlabach in a much-improved version of the rugged lodge a mountain family had lived in decades before, now called Homestead.[33] Six others were living in the community at the time.[34] I found that spending my days with people who had long histories with my dad opened doors to storytelling and conversations about him, which, if you believe in mystery as I do, may have kept his spirit alive among the trees.

"I think Nelson spent half his life on the phone," Bob Sabath told me once. Bob, who himself was on the phone just about every time I stopped by, moved to Rolling Ridge with his wife Jackie in 2002, largely because of conversations they'd had with Dad.

Bob was right. Whatever the project or community Dad was constructing, he used the telephone, and then e-mail, as a carpenter might use hammer and nails. These were his tools for making ideas come to life. People knew that if they answered the phone and heard Dad's voice, he was probably going to give them a job to do. And when they told these stories at his funeral, their groans were mixed with laughter and a deep satisfaction: When Dad gave you a job to do, it was as though he was handing you a certificate of appreciation that read, "I notice you. I affirm you. You are really good at what you do, and you can make a difference right here, right now."

And so it is that through affirmation of many individual gifts, Dad again and again nudged people into pitching in for the sake of a larger vision.

"But with Nelson," Bob continued, then paused, eyes suddenly swept with emotion. "With Nelson, it was never just business. When he called to ask you about something related to Rolling Ridge, or whatever project he was working on, he always did it with a genuine and personal touch. He wanted to know how you were doing, how things were going in your life."

Dad reflected sometimes on the difference between community-building and friendship-making. He claimed he was remarkably good at the first and not remotely good at the latter.

Even though my temptation would be to argue that Dad was just being modest, he may actually be right. There is a subtle line between friend-relationships and community-relationships, and I think Dad felt the distinction in real ways. Beyond his relationship with my mom, who was his best friend, most of Dad's social interaction revolved around a vision, a project, a joint work of creation—as described in each chapter of this book. Again and again, Dad brought people together for committee meetings, group discussions, and youth retreats, but he rarely met up with friends for coffee or a movie. In all the years I knew him, he never left for "a fishing weekend with the guys," or "a night out with the boys."

Still, people loved my dad because of the interest he took in every individual he encountered. If a child answered his phone call, he would make sure she told him something about school or her most recent soccer game before he asked to speak with her dad or mom. My college roommates grew accustomed to answering Dad's questions about their lives whenever they happened to answer his calls for me.

The cumulative effect of Dad's thoughtful interweaving of *business* and *personal touch*, as Bob put it, was that by the time Dad was struck with cancer at sixty, countless people would gladly have rioted in the streets to keep him alive. By that point, it was irrelevant whether they were his friend-friends or community-friends. As Bob reflected with me about Dad a full two years after his death, Bob's eyes teared up, his throat caught, and I very much doubted whether the distinction Dad made between friend- and community-making really mattered at all.

♣

I had goals for my summer at Rolling Ridge—the completion of this manuscript among them—but really, what led me to the mountains was something less concrete. It began as a seed Bob planted in my mind nearly a year earlier. When I couldn't shake the idea, it slowly grew into a personal yearning for silence and solitude.

Living at Rolling Ridge meant a drastic change of pace and scenery. I moved from inner-city Philadelphia and a neighborhood block of easily two hundred to a tract of land with many more deer than people. I had to learn to live differently.

I did a little teaching in town but mostly spent my days on the land, awaking many mornings without an alarm—something I never did in the city—writing, and taking long walks through the woods. I worked regularly in the garden, digging holes into the mountain clay, laying in compost. As my days passed un-harried, I began to notice—just as countless poets and songwriters before me—the small things of life: the way the dogwood blooms disappear before the mountain laurel show their faces, the way the whippoorwill strikes up its song at dusk, sometimes singing well into the darkness. I learned to step into my days like open fields, to be quiet, idle, and alone, and not be afraid of any of the three.

And everywhere I went, I found Dad's footprints: in the old cook shed, the cottage where we had once lived, the Retreat House; in the paths he helped clear and the people who live in the community.

Rolling Ridge's familiar paths, roads, and power lines began to knit themselves into a map in my head, just as I, bit by bit, pieced together my own quilt of loss and hope. The quiet space in my life was, though hard at times, a gift. When the summer ended and I left it for the noise of graduate school and city living, I went accompanied by voices I rediscovered in my more solitary life among the trees: a fierce whisper of inner stillness, the deep self-acceptance Dad had encouraged in me, and a gentle hum of divine and unconditional love.

Father's Voice
Study, Retreat, Community

There is a part of me that has never felt like a city person, even after more than three decades in Washington. I was born in the living room of my parents' farmhouse and grew up milking cows and swimming in the creek. Today, in the Blue Ridge Mountains of West Virginia, there is a place that has been part of my life for nearly thirty years, allowing me to stay connected with the land in ways that are hard to maintain in the city. The land is wooded and rugged, brown and green, and it is home to the Rolling Ridge Study Retreat Community.

Recently, a mother came to visit me and expressed how much her young son loves Rolling Ridge, how disappointed he was that he could not attend his Sunday school retreat there this past spring. It was so good to hear that this young, city-raised boy felt such a strong relationship to Rolling Ridge. Some urban families maintain privately owned beach homes and mountain cabins, where they can go for breaks from city life. My hope has been that Rolling Ridge could serve a similar purpose, allowing families to hold a connection to a piece of land outside the city—and to the larger natural world—without the financial burden of owning and maintaining it themselves.

Here I am not going to give a thorough history of Rolling Ridge's development. I want only to tell about my experience—about why Betty and I became involved and why Rolling Ridge, more than any other project I have worked on, has been so dear to me, so full of blessing and, at times, of overwhelming anxiety and difficulty.

__*Origins*__

During our young adult years, the fact that Betty and I didn't have children as soon as we could have allowed us more time and energy for other involvements. Our house at 2720 Ontario Road had a large front room which lent itself to gatherings and meetings. The space, along with other friends' living rooms and dining room tables, became vehicles for creative activity.

In the early seventies, a number of our friends began discussing the possibility of creating an intentional community in the country—an idea common in the sixties. Verle and Vivian Headings were key in this exploratory process, hosting periodic meetings in their home.[35] Betty and I were on the fringes of these conversations, as we did not have serious interest in leaving the city, but we shared many of the commitments and values being discussed. The group was on the lookout for land. I remember taking a trip down to the Charlottesville area with some of them to look at a piece of farmland and pasture as a possible location for their envisioned community.

Back in D.C., the Headings continued to host meetings, but it would be some time before a solid and committed group would develop. The circle of interested folks continued to form, change, and reform, along with the group's vision, which was growing to include not only intentional community but a weaving of three strands: community, study, *and* retreat.[36]

Sometime around 1974, the Headings learned about a property in West Virginia owned by Henry and Mary-Cushing Niles. This elderly Quaker couple planned to create a foundation to which they would bequeath roughly half of their mostly wooded acres.[37] They were interested in leasing parcels of the foundation land to groups developing projects that were ecumenical in nature, with strong communal and humanitarian commitments. Verle wrote an initial letter to the Niles about the possibility of building an intentional study-retreat community on some of the land.

In spring 1975, a group of us—five or six couples and families—went to see the land for ourselves. For one weekend, we stayed out along Route 9 at the Blue Ridge Campground, which has since closed down. At the time, the area was quite isolated, and I remember one member of the group, in particular, deciding that there was no way she would ever live out there in the "boonies."

While we were there, Verle made arrangements for us to meet with the Niles, who were staying in their summer home on the land. We walked around what was then an almost entirely wooded area before sitting down to talk with them. Following this trip, Verle drew up a proposal for a community retreat project and shared it with all of us and with the Niles couple, who took interest in our ideas.

__The Move to West Virginia__

Gradually, the group gathering regularly at the Headings home thinned down until only four couples were meeting: Verle and Vivian Headings, Paul and Ellen Peachey, Dabney and Alta Miller, and Betty and myself. The eight of us became the core members of the effort.

We had good ideas, but, as I remember it, we were stalled. We weren't sure how to make such a big leap from the city to the country, from Washington, D.C., to Jefferson County, West Virginia. Amid our quandary, a young man named Randy Tremba arrived in the D.C. area.[38] He shared our group's interest in community and, partly because his life was in transition at the time, he made an offer that changed the course of the Rolling Ridge story: He told us that he would go "spy out the land."

Randy moved to Jefferson County, West Virginia, and found a job as an orchard hired hand. He reported to the rest of us that we should consider moving to Shepherdstown, a small college town about forty-five minutes from Rolling Ridge, which, he said, wouldn't be as jarring as moving directly to the undeveloped ridge but would allow the group to be closer to it. On Randy's recommendation, Dabney, Alta, Verle, Vivian, and their children decided to move to Shepherdstown in 1975.[39]

The core members continued to meet regularly. Once a month, Paul, Ellen, Betty, and I would drive out to Shepherdstown; or Verle, Vivian, Dabney, and Alta would make the trip into the city.

The following year, the eight of us, along with our families, Randy Tremba, and a few other friends, arranged to do a whole week of overnight tent-camping on the land. There were thirty of us in all. In 1976, the place we now call Rolling Ridge was mostly wilderness. A jeep trail led to a clearing[40] where we parked our cars and then walked into the woods a short distance to find spots for our tents. While we were there, we used logs and heavy canvas to build our first structure on the land—what we called a cook tent.

Our camping group divided into four teams and went out to explore different sections of the land, using maps. The total tract included mountainside, flatter formerly farmed young forest, and a descent to the Shenandoah River. We wrote down notes about what we discovered, giving particular attention to whether this land could lend itself to building a community. Through those explorations, we identified a section of land for which we would apply to the Niles for a lease. Our preferred piece of land included two hillsides with a stream running between them. We hoped to develop a live-in community on one side of the ravine and retreat facilities on the other—as is true today.

The week of camping was a significant time for all of us. Then, in 1977, our group was leased 130 acres of the Niles' foundation land for our envisioned community and retreat center.[41] According to the forty-year lease, redone in 1997, the foundation owns the land, which it "rents" to the Rolling Ridge Study Retreat Community for free.

Interestingly, among the four couples in the core group, only Betty and I had no declared interest in living on the land. We all anticipated that the other three couples would move to the land over the next several years and develop the project further—and that by 1980, we would have a great deal accomplished. In reality, everything took much longer than we had thought.

__Molding a Vision__

Even though Betty and I did not plan to move to Rolling Ridge with the Headings, Peacheys, and Millers, we were becoming more deeply involved in the dreaming.

My interest in the project was growing. I didn't have a strong understanding of "retreat"—which along with "study" and "community" made up the three strands of our vision. I *was* excited by the concept of shared space and resources. I was interested in the notion of communities and cooperatives—people working together to create expanded options for themselves—and it was those aspects of the vision for Rolling Ridge, as well as my love of the land, that motivated me to stay involved.

Why do people get stuck on needing high incomes? I would ask myself. I believed it was possible to live on considerably less money by sharing with others to satisfy some of one's wants. I imagined city families coming to Rolling Ridge and, in so doing, building community rather than cultivating the individualism that was becoming more and more common throughout society. Thus, Rolling Ridge would not only give families a connection to open space and land outside the city but also allow them to live on lower incomes and participate in a larger vision, something beyond themselves.

At our monthly meetings, we talked about what Rolling Ridge could be and how to get there. Would we plant an orchard or have a farm? Would community members work mostly on the land—or would they hold off-site jobs to support themselves?

And what kind of houses would we build? I liked the idea of a cooperative housing arrangement, in which families would live in homes clustered very close together—or even in one building—sharing certain household spaces. One large building would be more energy efficient than individual houses, all exposed to the elements.

I, however, was alone in my vision for cooperative housing. Most of the others—the people who were actually going to live at Rolling Ridge—wanted the residential community to be spread out.

♣

We had challenges and differences within the group over other aspects of the Rolling Ridge vision as well. One of the first issues we faced had to do with a local West Virginia family that was already living on the land we had leased from the Niles.

In 1976 when we toured the land, we learned that the Jones family, an older couple with a young son, were living in a small cottage on the hillside where we hoped to develop the live-in community. Their cottage was very simple with no plumbing, so they carried water up from the stream. They had an informal relationship with the Niles, who allowed them to live on the land and take some responsibility for overseeing the property, but legally, they had no lease to the land.

Did we have a right to ask them to leave? Legally, we did, but was it ethical to displace an underprivileged family? There was a lot of ambiguity and ambivalence about whether or how to get them to move from the land or who would do it. It was a sensitive and moral issue that brought out differences among us, so it took more than a year to make a decision. In the end, we did ask the Jones family to leave but did so with as much care as possible. They moved to a small house on a property they owned a few miles away.

I also remember animated differences over whether to file for tax-exempt 501(c)(3) status. Dabney felt strongly that becoming a tax-exempt organization would tie us into a larger system we didn't believe in because of our opposition to war—

the American tax system. Others believed this was a necessary step in developing our community and retreat program. Despite Dabney's hesitations, we did eventually achieve 501(c)(3) status, but not until 1985.

Beyond this, we also discussed how much this project would be involved in the local Blue Ridge community, rather than being tied only to people from the D.C. metropolitan area. And would Rolling Ridge benefit strictly the middle class, or could it also serve the poor?

We talked and talked, to the extent that after a while, it felt like we were just spinning our wheels. The key question in my mind became this: How were we going to get moving on this thing and assemble the resources to make it work? Slowly, we did make some decisions and progress, though I think we were all a bit overwhelmed by the daunting size of the vision we wished to bring to life.

__Living on the Land__

We made some headway on plans for the residential community in the early 1980s. We spent a weekend with someone who had architectural training and land-use-planning experience and developed the idea of having the historic garden wall serve as the center hub of the community. This wall also formed one wall of the Jones family's small cottage, which nestled against the hillside. Other houses would form a crescent along the hillside around the wall. Lots were drawn up. Verle did much of the work involved in creating a plan that was then presented to the county for approval. The Headings, Peacheys, and Millers all came up with proposed homes. Still, it was years before any of these couples moved to the land.

A fifth couple were the first to live at Rolling Ridge. Jay and Marilyn Good became involved in the early '80s. They and their family had just returned from a Peace Corps term in Latin America and lived in Annville, Pennsylvania. I helped recruit them to move to Rolling Ridge in 1981. Jay and Marilyn did not mind primitive conditions, so Jay and Dabney built additional bedrooms onto the back of the small, rustic cottage where the Jones family had lived, and the young family moved in.

We all had these big dreams. Jay and Marilyn Good were interested in living in community, which is largely what drew them to Rolling Ridge. We expected that, with the help of Jay's skills in construction and carpentry, we would soon build other homes on the hillside, and that the Headings, Peacheys, and Millers would join Jay and Marilyn in the intentional community we had envisioned.

In actuality, development was much slower. The Peacheys' house didn't get underway until 1985. Jay served as construction foreman, but in the end, Jay, Marilyn, and their children decided to leave Rolling Ridge in 1986, shortly before the Peacheys moved into their new home.

♣

In the early 1980s, Betty and I were juggling family life, Learning Center, and WSSY involvements. With two and then three small children, it became more and more difficult to get to the group's monthly meetings, and Betty started questioning her relationship to Rolling Ridge. I continued attending regularly and Betty as often as she could, until eventually Betty formally withdrew her commitment from the core group.

Amid this family transition and my own questions about vocation and life goals, however, we decided to move to Rolling Ridge for five months, from May to October 1982. In doing so, we were modeling one of my visions for Rolling Ridge—that it be a place where people can go for sabbatical-type experiences.

The one-room cottage where our family would live was simply an outer wall with open studs. Before we moved, I made day-trips out to Rolling Ridge to work with Jay in improving the cottage, adding insulation and closing it up. The cottage had no electricity. We used battery and oil lamps, got up with the sun, and went to bed when it got dark. At first, we also had no water. Jay rigged up a fifty-five-gallon tank up the hill from the cottage, which would flow by gravity down to us to give us cold water from a sink. We also put in a gas stove and a gas refrigerator. In the end, it was a very livable space.

Betty and I hoped to use the summer to reflect on our being in the city. At the time, I was splitting my time between the FLOC Learning Center and Washington Study-Service Year. I wondered about branching out in a new way, possibly pursuing more education. I already had a Masters in Sociology from the early '70s, but I remember considering teaching or pursuing a degree in business as well, so that I could be a more professional administrator of organizations.

If we were going to stay in the city long term, I thought it was a good idea to spend a period of time looking at it from the outside. It also seemed more likely that we would stay in the city if we had a chance to get away, which I think was true. So, all in all, it was a very fruitful summer for us.

Jay and Marilyn's family were living on the other side of the ravine. They were meeting for supper once a week with the Shepherdstown community, and during our family's sabbatical we became part of the group as well. The Peacheys were still in D.C. but came out for meetings once a month.

At Rolling Ridge, Jay and I worked together on a number of projects, and friends came out for work camps. We changed the cook tent into a cook shed, which still stands, rotting out, on its original site, and we made improvements to the ten-sided dome where we held many of our meetings. Our core group was also running wilderness retreats on various themes; participants stayed in tents, as we did not yet have any retreat facilities. We built canvas and pole structures to protect individual campsites. It was a good summer, a dynamic time.

__*A Place for Retreats*__

I tried to think of ways to fund the construction of houses and retreat facilities at Rolling Ridge. As we developed our vision, we didn't want to be obligated by loans on program-related facilities. These buildings, I thought, should be debt-free. We decided that we would construct all program-related facilities only with charitable gifts. Community houses, on the other hand, could be built using loan money, which would be paid off in the coming years with rent paid by the community members. The community members would all live in rental houses owned by Rolling Ridge Study Retreat and sitting on land owned by the Niles' Rolling Ridge foundation.

We continued to brainstorm about our vision for a retreat program. Paul had lots of ideas for Rolling Ridge becoming a significantly academic setting, a study center. Over the years, Verle in particular has held on to this hope as a critical part of our vision, an idea that stands in some tension with others' notion of retreat as primarily contemplative.

Today, unless someone really stirs up old documents, I think we all remember the original vision for retreat facilities differently. In my memory, we envisioned a central building that would be a conference center of sorts, with a library and study and the capacity to serve food to large groups but with no bedding. It would have big windows facing the clearing, with a nice view of the mountain. Three or four smaller retreat cottages, spread across the hillside, would provide lodging for those attending larger retreats or serve as private hermitages for individuals or small groups on personal retreats.

These were ambitious plans, and by the late 1980s, after Paul and Ellen had been living on the land for about a year, we still had not begun any construction on the retreat side of the ravine. I began to feel that a conference center *and* cottages were just too big an undertaking. Doing it all at once would be impossible, considering our limited resources, yet building just a conference center did not make sense without also building the cottages to support it.

I began to push for a compromise. I thought, *We've got to get something going, or we need to shut up and pack out.* We had already put a lot of resources into building Paul and Ellen's house. So I became the primary generator of a middle-ground proposal—that we would construct one building with modest sleeping, gathering, and eating accommodations: the Retreat House.

♣

How would we fund the construction of the Retreat House? I started advancing the idea of "partner groups." The partner groups I envisioned would be mostly Washington-area congregations who would buy into the project and then, in return, have reserved use of the Retreat House a certain number of weekends every year. Partner groups would buy "shares" at the outset, helping to fund the building. These shares could later be sold back to Rolling Ridge should they choose to do so, allowing Rolling Ridge to sell them to other groups. Partner groups would also pay an annual operating fee, adjusted each year based on the cost of maintaining the facility.

In a more common retreat center model, the center provides and advertises retreats, for which individuals sign up to participate and pay registration fees. At Rolling Ridge, as it has turned out, we usually plan six to ten activities a year that fit this model. But during the other forty-some weekends, partner groups use the Retreat House for their own activities.

Currently, partner groups plan a variety of retreats, often using resource people from their own congregations rather than paying someone else to come in. In this way, Rolling Ridge creates a place where small churches can have a retreat facility without building one themselves or hustling to rent something. They are guaranteed the space every year, which in turn encourages them to build a retreat rhythm into their own congregational life.

It is a great arrangement in the sense that partner groups' annual fees cover the cost of operating the Retreat House from year to year, while the retreats and activities they plan for themselves save Rolling Ridge the large overhead costs involved in marketing and running retreats week after week.[42]

The partner-group structure allowed us to pull together resources for building the Retreat House and then to operate it in a sustainable way without crippling overhead costs. I think it was one of my significant contributions to Rolling Ridge.

__Fundraising__

Before we started construction on the Retreat House, I presented the idea of partner groups to the core members of Rolling Ridge and the recently formed board for their approval and then started recruiting partner groups. I think it was 1986.

I still had many connections in the city from my earlier work with voluntary service and then, more recently, in placing WSSY students in internships. I began talking to the network of people I knew, the churches, organizations, and individuals—all of this on volunteer time. Early on in the effort, Luther Place, a large Lutheran church on 14th Street, came through big time, buying five shares.

Gradually, my list of partner groups grew. I relied on relationships and trust. I guess people would say, "Well, Nelson's a good guy. It sounds like he has a good idea. Let's just go with it." Without the trust and connections I had built in the city, the partner group development would have been much more difficult.

We began construction of the Retreat House before I had committed partner groups for all of the available shares, but in the end, we sold nineteen shares to ten partner groups. Each share was worth two weekends at the Retreat House. And we kept six shares (twelve weekends) for retreats planned by the Rolling Ridge community and board.

Recruiting the partner groups brought together a pile of funds, but I knew, based on our budget, that it wouldn't be enough. Before starting construction, I wanted to raise another $20,000 in donations. I hoped to raise half of that through

$1,000 contributions. I didn't consider myself a fundraiser and had very little experience, but I did what I knew how to do: I talked to people who knew me.

I remember paying a visit to one man in particular some-time early in the fundraising effort. He was a well-established man and a friend to Paul and Ellen Peachey through Hyattsville Mennonite Church. I met with him in his living room; I think it was a Sunday afternoon. I was hoping he would give me some ideas for how to raise this money, and more than that, that he would contribute some of his own.

He suggested some ideas, but it became clear to me that he wasn't prepared to carry much weight. I remember feeling like I was almost begging him. I was so desperate to get these funds together. "Would you help me get started with a significant gift?" I asked.

He was hesitating, but I told him, "You know, I wouldn't be doing this except for Paul and Ellen Peachey. They built this house and moved out to Rolling Ridge in good faith that we would be developing this project. And in good faith, I'm doing my best to see that we make the next step." I was making it sound like some great moral duty.

And he said, "Well, I'll help with a thousand dollars." It wasn't enough to knock me over, but it was the first real step of affirmation. This man's thousand was followed by others. Betty's brother and father came through, as did a cousin who gave a thousand dollars and made me promise that I would never come back to ask for more.

Again, people did not give money because they knew any-thing about the Rolling Ridge project. And in most cases, they would never benefit from it. People gave money because of my—or Paul Peachey's—personal relationships with them. Fi-nally, even though there were still several shares that needed to be sold to partner groups, we determined we had enough money to begin construction.

__*The Concrete Nightmare*__

When our family was on our sabbatical, back in 1982, I remember traipsing around Rolling Ridge, beginning to imagine a retreat house and where we could build it. This was before we had discussed it at length in the group. I remember later being amazed how long it took to turn the idea into reality.

I left the Learning Center in December 1986 and WSSY in June 1987. My decision to leave was not only driven by the need for change in those organizations but also partly by the pressing need for leadership in developing the Retreat House at Rolling Ridge. I devoted much of 1988 to fulltime work on the building. It became its own chapter in my life because it developed into such an all-consuming project. There was some pay, but cash was short. Funding was a real problem. Because I controlled where the money went, I don't think I paid myself very much.

In constructing the Retreat House, our Rolling Ridge group made a number of compromises in our ideals. We hoped, as much as possible, to use stone and wood from the land in the construction of buildings on the land. Some of the residential houses have stuck more closely to this ideal. Because time seemed really important, however, the Retreat House was built with a concrete-block foundation and bought lumber that was not from the land. We used rough-cut wood from a local sawmill for the siding. And due to our tight budget, we used particle board and plywood in some of the construction, which is not as environmentally friendly because glues in these materials can release toxins into the air.

I recruited David Conrad, an architectural student I knew, to do basic drawings. A committee reviewed a plan for the design of the Retreat House, and then David put it to paper. We had a bulldozer clear the land at the site, creating big piles of trees and stumps, with hopes of getting the footers put in by May.

It was a terribly wet spring. We just could not get the footers we dug to stay dry, because springs kept coming out at different places. We actually had to shift the site of the Retreat House about five feet from where David had planned it because we ran into so much water.

We did eventually get it dry enough to set in rebar and get everything prepared to pour the concrete. Then it rained *again,* and I ended up digging mud from around the rebar by myself with a shovel. It was just dreadful.

♣

We finally thought we were ready for the concrete. The night before the trucks were scheduled to come, I stayed at Paul and Ellen Peachey's house on the land. I hardly slept, worrying about getting the trucks in the rough, dirt roads because the ground was so soft from all the rain. My memory is that we had eleven inches of rain in one month, which just saturated the mountain.

When the two truckers arrived the next day, I showed them the route I had planned to take them to the Retreat House site, but they said, "No way. We can't get in there." They asked if there was any other way, so I showed them a possibility they agreed to try. It involved going up toward the clearing, turning left, and coming down the hill toward the Retreat House.

The first truck went in, with the other guy giving directions, but he just couldn't make the turn off the road going up to the clearing. When he tried to back himself out, he got stuck against a tree. I could see we were in trouble. I made a decision early on that—expensive as it was—we were going to have to dump the concrete somewhere in the woods, that there was no way we could get in to the site.

We were working against the clock because the concrete would set up in the trucks. One of the drivers was a strong guy who could really run a chain saw. He had to get the tree cut and thrown and the stump cut down low enough so that the stuck mixer's tires could roll by. The tree fell against the truck, which he then rocked so that it actually threw the tree away from the mixer. I think we may have had a tractor and a rope pulling at the same time.

Only Tom Donlon, our master builder, was there to help me, because Paul and Ellen had gone to a wedding. It was enormously stressful for me. We did succeed in getting the trucks to a place where I had decided to dump the concrete, sort of hidden in the woods, off to the side of the road. As the second truck dumped its concrete, we could see it coming out in big clumps; it was that close to hardening. Thankfully, I don't think there was damage to either truck.

Sometime after that incident, my dad called and we talked about it on the phone. Then he said, "How much does a share cost?"

"Twenty-six hundred," I told him.[43]

"I'll send you a check for $2,600," he said. "And I want you to keep it yourself."

♣

In that one nightmare of an experience, it seemed the whole project was close to falling through. And much of the problem was that I was in over my head. I was working with a tight budget, trying to save money, but my lack of experience was showing everywhere. I knew, for example, that we would eventually need to make a new road into the Retreat House, but I now know that on a project like this, I should have created access first, not later.

How was I going to get the concrete company to come in again after the first almost-catastrophe? I remember a day or two after the crisis, standing with Verle, Dabney, Paul, and a local excavator named Claude "Buddy" Marcum, discussing the problem. "Well," we said, "we're going to have to build a new road, even though it will cost us considerable money."

Marcum, the excavator, knew the land very well and knew where there had once been a road, so we had him build a new one, wide enough for a truck. Then he convinced the concrete company that he would have his tractors there prepared to pull a truck through if necessary. The road he built is today the lane into the Retreat House.

__Building the Retreat House__

I spent 1988 as the general contractor for the construction of the Retreat House, and I was learning on the job. Tom Donlon was the carpenter, the actual builder for the project, and he was key in that he had a fair amount of experience in building. Other subcontractors came in with their specialties. I recruited Byron Marsh to do the electrical work and plumbing for a song. And I recruited some volunteers to help Tom over the summer.

There were many challenges. I had a hard time finding a site for the sewage drainage field. You need a drainage field that perks at an approved rate to get a building permit from the county. And we just couldn't get adequate perk. I worked and worked, testing so many different holes. That was driving me crazy that spring.

I felt at times that we just muddled through the project, sometimes literally—like when Buddy Marcum and I were running the water line from the pump house up to the Retreat House. We had to take the line under the spring at the bottom of the ravine, but the large plastic pipe wanted to float—it wouldn't stay down. We didn't want to put heavy rocks on it because eventually they would break the thing, but we had to anchor it somehow.

I got in the water and stood on the pipe while Marcum gradually scooped buckets of ground on top. I fished rocks out to make sure they wouldn't break the pipe. Bit by bit we got it to stay down, with the stream still flowing over top. I was in with mud up to my waist; it was one big mess. Afterward, Marcum made some comment about "rarely seeing *that* side of what a general contractor does." He was so impressed, he gave me a gift of vegetables from his garden. And he wasn't a guy to appreciate educated people at all.

♣

There were times I wondered if the Retreat House was not going to happen. But we were already committed in so many ways. It's hard to pull out after personal effort and resources have already been invested, with Paul and Ellen living out on the land and partner groups committed with their money.

And why had this become my project? I can't remember exactly, but there must have been an evolutionary process of sorts. We sorely needed a retreat house, and our group was not sure how to make it happen. Betty remembers that early in the process, it was she who spoke up in a meeting, saying I was the one most suited for the job. She believed fully in my abilities as a leader, but I'm sure she had no idea of the toll it would later take on our relationship.

I estimated in the budget that the project would pay me a modest amount for a certain number of hours of my time. And I remember Alta Miller saying, "You're crazy. There's no way we're going to do it in those few hours." She was right. I dumped in hours upon hours that year.

♣

I remember another story about how close I came to making a mistake in the construction of the Retreat House. Tom Donlon, the builder, had worked carefully at putting up the beams that are visible when you walk into the Retreat House. One Saturday, when I had a bunch of volunteers helping, I had to come up with jobs for them to do. I had just given instructions to several volunteers to paint those beams white.

Tom came to me and explained that it was his understanding the whole time that we would put only a clear finish on the beams, preserving their natural color. "I wouldn't have put so much time and care into them," he said, "if I had known they were just going to be painted over."

"Oh!" I said. "I didn't realize that. Let's stop right now." Thankfully, the volunteers hadn't started painting. That would have been such a serious mistake, because everybody who comes to the Retreat House now talks about how beautiful those beams are. If they had been painted white, the space would be far less attractive, and it would have been hard to strip them down.

It was providential, in my book, that Tom overheard me, and that he had the thoughtfulness to say something to me. As general contractor, it was really my decision whether or not to paint beams, and Tom could have decided, *Well, that's his problem*. But he asserted himself. I am so glad he did.

By the end of 1988, we had the Retreat House mostly finished. We were short on workers and ran out of money, so a few things were not completed when the first group came for a retreat New Year's weekend. The porch deck and the screened in porch weren't put on, and the drainage field for the septic system was not installed. These were all completed by the following summer, thanks to the help of a number of folks, including that year's WSSY students.

__Reflections__

What is amazing to me about the Retreat House is that we got stuck with only one. I thought we'd build a second, similar facility soon afterward because a number of churches were interested in taking larger groups out for retreats. I always told them we'd have a second one built in four or five years. But today, more than fifteen years later, that still has not happened. It says something about how hard it was to do a project like this. Today the Rolling Ridge community and board still discuss building a second retreat house, but there is considerable uncertainty about it.

I learned a lot from my year working on the Retreat House, particularly about fundraising and construction. I had done a little construction growing up on the farm, and Betty and I had done a total renovation job on our first house on Ontario Road in Adams Morgan, but I had never done anything like this before. It astonishes me now to look back at projects I took on in my life, and I wonder why I was so willing to risk doing them without much experience.

It was quite a hard year, and I felt alone at times. Very alone. Paul was a strong moral presence; I could talk to him and feel his support. There were others from the core group and friends like Marlin Good from in town who helped to make it happen, but no one was helping me solve problems on a day-to-day basis.

The stress of getting the Retreat House completed put pressure on our family life. I put in long hours, often getting up early in the morning to go out to Rolling Ridge (about one and a half hours away) and coming back late at night. Sometimes I would stay out overnight working on the project. As a result, I was not very available to Betty nor to our three children. I think I even missed the annual family beach trip that year. I was much more absent from the family than ever before or since, and Betty felt deserted.

I remember sitting in the kitchen at home, and Betty was sharing some of her frustrations. "I feel caught," I told her. "I have to see this thing through."

In a burst of emotion I added, "I hope no one ever thanks me for getting this retreat house done. If they want to be supportive, *now* is the time to be here for me. If they really appreciated it, they would have been here when it hurt!" I don't know exactly what I said. I think I cursed. I was just so angry and felt so alone, and the project was demanding so much, to the extent that my wife was upset with me.

In January 1989, House Church had its first retreat at the Retreat House. It was a nice large group at worship Sunday morning. I forget the nature and structure of the worship, but during sharing time, Betty talked about how hard it was for her to be at Rolling Ridge. The Retreat House had come to represent to her a "mistress"—*my* mistress because it had taken me away from her. She shared this in tears.

That was hard for me to hear and made me wish deeply that I had found a way to have managed the project while being more available to my family. It was a point of learning. I think over the years since, we have mostly healed. But the Retreat House was not done without grief and stress.

__The Years Since__

After the Retreat House was built, I thought we needed to focus only on fundraising and plans for new facilities that would enhance the use of the house. Paul Peachey thought we needed someone to write the story of Rolling Ridge up through 1990, and I thought he was wrong. There were much more important things to be spending our time and money on. But Paul got the board to approve Tom Donlon to write the history.

Now, in hindsight, I see how valuable that writing project was and is. The booklet, *The Faith Road to Rolling Ridge*, sustains the memory of Rolling Ridge, which is important because otherwise, it would soon be lost. Paul and Ellen Peachey are now in a retirement community and aren't directly involved with Rolling Ridge anymore. Dabney and Alta decided to move to Virginia, detaching from the core group. Betty is only peripherally involved, and I am dying.

Of the original core members, only Verle and Vivian are still involved and hold the long-term memory of the place. Donlon's writing helped preserve the core group's thread of vision, even as the people involved in Rolling Ridge have changed. I am now grateful for Paul's foresight.[44]

Ellen Peachey had the vision and leadership to start the Meditative Arts Program, a committee that sponsors two retreats a year. They wanted a facility outside of the Retreat House for doing art activities, so they helped raise money to fix up the cottage where we had stayed for our sabbatical and transformed it into what we now call the Art Cottage. They painted the inside walls and made the space much more attractive, complete with tables, cabinets, and art supplies.

A second project in the late 1990s was the building of the Meditation Shelter. Here again I didn't have a lot of interest, and I thought we should instead put our energy toward building a second retreat house or hermitage—because I thought we needed to create additional lodging for overnight retreats.

Paul Peachey, though, had the vision for building a meditation shelter as a small chapel and a symbol of Rolling Ridge's commitment to meditation. It would have ten sides, like the base of the plastic-covered geodesic dome we had built more than ten years earlier for meetings. We would build it where the dome once sat, as another way of preserving the history and memory of the place.

Building the Meditation Shelter took time and effort, but people love it. It's beautiful, a lovely place to go for prayer and for meetings outside the Retreat House.

♣

My role at Rolling Ridge has been unique in that no one else has had my level of involvement and *not* been part of the residential community. In some senses, I am considered halfway part of the community because of my history in the original core group. That has given me a certain legitimacy and influence even though I am, technically, just a long-term volunteer.

I think I was only on the Rolling Ridge board as a voting member for its first six years (1985-1991), but the by-laws prevented me from staying on more than six years in a row. Ever since, I have been an "ad hoc" (non-voting) board member, sitting in on meetings and volunteering to be on committees, agreeing to work with this person or that person in getting something done.

Other than the years when I was a board member, I haven't had a formal position at Rolling Ridge. Generally, I would say I have been a supportive presence to many efforts at Rolling Ridge, often giving hours of my time, occasionally rearranging my work schedule to make that possible, and sometimes having significant influence in decision-making. The informality of my role has left the door open for misunderstandings, but my involvements have been, for the most part, endorsed by the board.

In the years since completing the Retreat House, I have done many different things: some administrative tasks, some manual labor, some project coordination. I have managed the schedule for the use of the Retreat House and worked closely with Ellen and then Vivian in overseeing its upkeep and care. I have generally helped shape ideas, recruit volunteers, and organize work camps. I put in a lot of time building the Meditation Shelter.

I have done the tax reports each year and overseen the financial management of the organization, doing the analysis of our costs and revenue. And my network of relationships has been crucial in fundraising, recruiting partner groups, and shaping the community of people who have finally chosen to live out at Rolling Ridge.

__Rolling Ridge Today__

In the past two years, the network of people invested in Rolling Ridge has shifted and expanded. They have kept Rolling Ridge's threads of study and retreat viable and alive, even as the residential community members have changed.

Today, Pinestone, the house Paul and Ellen Peachey built and lived in for many years, is used as retreat space for individuals and small groups, or as spill-over space when large groups use the Retreat House. The Peacheys lived at Rolling Ridge for about fifteen years before moving to a retirement community in Virginia.

Verle and Vivian Headings lived in Shepherdstown and then in an old summer cottage nearby that belonged to the Niles, while they built their house at Rolling Ridge. It was a slow process, because they used stones off the land to build the foundation, wood from trees on the land, and mostly volunteer labor. Meanwhile, Verle was very busy with his work at Howard University in Washington. After years of planning and effort, they finally moved into Deerspring, their beautiful home in the Rolling Ridge community, in 1999.

Keith Lyndaker had first been to Rolling Ridge as a WSSY student and simply liked the place. He returned to the city after graduating from college, but after a few years, found the city tired and overwhelming. He got this idea that he'd like to live out in West Virginia, wondering if he could figure out his next steps from there.

In 1992, we began working together on a plan for him to live in the old homestead (where Jay and Marilyn had once lived) for six months and work on various projects on the land. He moved out the following March. After six months, he extended his stay and then continued to extend it until he had become very attached. He has since married Rachelle Schlabach and fixed up Homestead, where they now live together.

Bob and Jackie Sabath are the third couple in the Rolling Ridge residential community. I first got to know them when Jackie was succeeding me as WSSY's coordinator. I remember traveling with both of them to an event at Eastern Mennonite College and talking with Bob about his interest in retreat ministry and community living.

Bob and I stayed in touch over the years, planning work camps, youth activities, and a boys club for our teenage children and church youth. I was thrilled when he and Jackie started talking about moving to Rolling Ridge more than five years ago. I was part of a committee that met with them regularly as they processed their decision. They built their house during 2000 and 2001 with the help of many friends and paid carpentry help, including Jay Good, and then moved out in February 2002.[45]

♣

Rolling Ridge is a testament to the ways that a vision can survive, even as people come and go from a community, organization, or project. I have a lot of confidence in the wide base of people who care about this special place in the Blue Ridge Mountains of West Virginia and hope that new folks with their vision and unique gifts will continue to be drawn there. I feel sure that Rolling Ridge will continue to provide a place for urban families and churches to connect with nature and each other, long after I'm gone.

may 11, 2005

Doctor Fojo, who knows more about ACC than almost anyone, is one of the most compassionate people I have met. He sits so close to my dad, their knees touch. Though Doctor Fojo has (and loses) dozens of patients every year, he feels to us almost a part of our family. We have depended on his knowledge and guidance over and over in the past two months. And though we like and trust him, the purpose of today's appointment has us feeling anxious—even fearful.

In an earlier visit, Doctor Fojo had assessed the severity of Dad's condition. He was candid: The situation did not look good. Not only was Dad's cancer rare, aggressive, and well-progressed, but it had spread to the bones, which only happens in a few ACC cases. "But I am not running up a white flag yet," he'd promised.

He had run through treatment options, explaining that there was no way to predict which treatment would be most likely to help an individual patient. To which Dad had smiled and responded, "So treatment's pretty much a crap shoot."

It is now two months later. Two rounds of cisplatin infusions later. Two bouts of extreme nausea and debilitating depression later. Dad has lost weight but, miraculously, not his hair.

A few days ago, we were at NIH for a CT-scan, and today we have returned for the results. Back in January, it was a CT-scan at Washington Hospital Center that rocked us irreversibly, showing an entirely unexpected tumor on Dad's left adrenal gland. Now, once again, a CT-scan will determine our future. Has the chemotherapy had any effect on the cancer? If not, how fast is the cancer progressing?

Doctor Fojo's answers are not easy to swallow.

When we arrive home from NIH, Mom feels depleted, inside-out. Dad's mind is gently sorting the news, but he too looks exhausted. Yet before we can crawl into our beds or take our walks or beat our pillows with our fists, we have a responsibility to which we must attend. As we have done, over and over since the diagnosis, we will let others into our circle—first and foremost, my two brothers. We call Ryan, who is between classes in Indiana, and e-mail Jason, who is traveling in Costa Rica.

Then, in the pair of the hour, as Mom reels and Dad rests, it becomes my job to share the news with all our friends and family, those who have surrounded and cared for us from the beginning, who will continue to do so in the weeks and months to come. I sit down at the computer and type an e-mail:[46]

Dear All,

Mom has been doing most of the writing recently, but tonight, I write for all of us. As many of you know, today was a significant day. On Monday, Dad, Mom, and I were at NIH for a CT-scan. And today, we were there again to meet with Dr. Fojo and his staff to learn what news the scan brought.

We arrived at NIH a little before our 12:30 appointment. Our physician friend, Dr. Brad Leissa, met us in the waiting room. We wondered at the fact that they even bother scheduling appointments—it was at least an hour and a half before they called Dad for a physical exam. Then, Brad and I joined Mom and Dad for the conference with Dr. Fojo.

The news was hard to hear. The CT-scan shows disease progression in Dad's lungs and liver. (There isn't significant progression in his bones.) Fojo expects the disease in Dad's liver to be what will eventually take his life. As the liver begins to fail, Dad will gradually get weaker and weaker.

Dad wanted to know how soon. Dr. Fojo said that he has no crystal ball. He said he chooses to give patients the worst case and then hope for the best. Worst case, he said, Dad has only one month to six weeks.

We were all shaken by how short it is.

Dr. Fojo's recommendations agree with our thinking: We are not pursuing any further treatment and will be stopping the mitotane. Dad will probably regain his appetite, the nausea will subside, and he will get stronger. He is also scheduled for a blood transfusion that will help boost his energy, which has been lagging. We will be pursuing hospice support right away.

Dr. Fojo and, later, Brad gave us more details about what to expect as his liver eventually loses function. They do not anticipate he will suffer much pain. For this, we are grateful.

The short prognosis definitely affects how we think about the next days, weeks, and months. We are still reeling a bit and aren't sure what to tell those of you who are also reeling and those who want to be supportive.

For now, we'll say this: We feel surrounded by love. Love can't always heal pain, but it helps heal loneliness. So thank you. With the great uncertainties of the immediate future, we are unsure how to manage phone calls, offers to visit with us, and offers to help in other ways. For now, please hang on to them and instead, plant a flower, light candles, make cookies with your kids. We will write again after we've talked further as a family about how we most want to spend our time and energy.

Love,
Deborah, for the rest

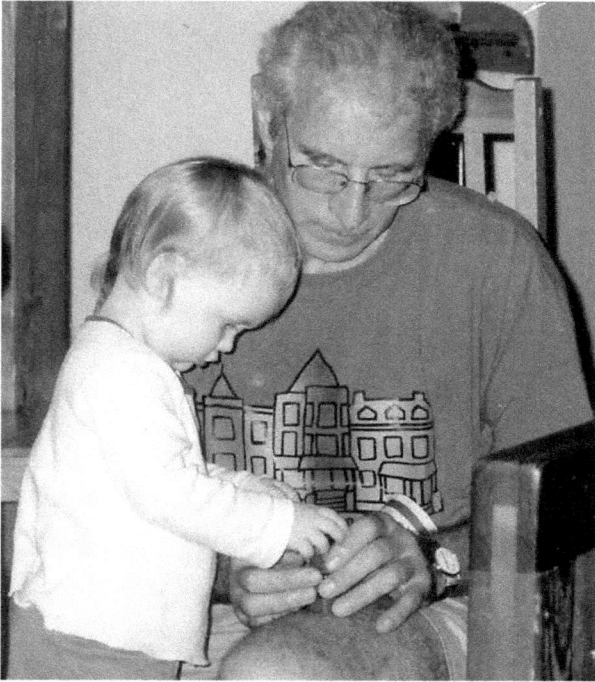

Nelson gives his full attention to the game he is playing with young Nora Charles at a House Church gathering. Photo credit: Dan Charles, 2000

Chapter 5

COMMUNITY
HOUSE CHURCH

Daughter's Voice
Swamp-Swimming

Before attending college and then moving into the troubled multiculturalism of Washington, D.C., Dad was a farm boy. He grew up among cows, conservative Mennonites, and a way of life steeped deeply in Pennsylvania Dutch culture and religious tradition. Ruth, his mother, wore a cape dress and head covering until the day she died. His father, Ira, was chosen by lot to serve as the minister at Hammer Creek Mennonite Church. Ira wore a plain coat and led the family in devotions every morning at breakfast.[47] Though I am rooted in this same history and culture, the world of my dad's childhood is one I will never fully experience, one I cannot adequately describe, one to which I will never truly belong.

I, on the other hand, grew up navigating city buses, multi-lingual schools, and the colorful cloud of pluralism. I was clear that my family and my church were made up of Christians, and that I was one of them. I found that our version of the faith made me feel different from even the Christians at the public schools my brothers and I attended. I also didn't understand what any of this had to do with my classmates and teachers who were Muslims, Buddhists, atheists, and, if Christians, sometimes half-Jewish at the same time.

I was a shy child-turned-adolescent, intimidated by the separateness I felt at school. My parents never drank alcohol, a lifestyle choice I tied closely to our Christian faith. We prayed before supper, attended church on Sundays, and believed in a countercultural, nonviolent Jesus.

I mostly kept these differences to myself and, if absolutely necessary, summed them up with a word none of my friends at school had ever heard before. I come from a *Mennonite* family, I'd tell them. They tried out the strange combination of syllables, catching them awkwardly on their unpracticed tongues. *Men-a-night.* Okay.[48]

In between my adolescent self-consciousness and my inability to make sense of the religious smorgasbord at school, there was Community House Church. The church felt like a safe place for me as a child, a place where adults loved me and believed in a God who loved me too. I didn't realize at the time how unique the church was—in its strong community focus, its openness to uncertainty and raw honesty, its resistance to doctrine—and how much I would come to appreciate those very aspects of its personality.

♣

Community House Church, commonly referred to simply as "House Church" by those who know it, began in the '70s in Washington's Mount Pleasant neighborhood as a supper group, which then grew into an ecumenical worshipping community. After spending time in two other churches, my parents joined the group in its early years, becoming members in 1978.

The small, informal church eventually outgrew living rooms and has met in a variety of locations since but has always maintained its homegrown ethos. It is unique in its lay-leadership structure and its independence from a larger institutional church.

A friend from my days as a Christian-summer-camper once went along with me to a Sunday morning worship service at House Church. I knew she had grown up attending a church with several hundred neatly dressed Mennonites and doing the usual Mennonite-church things: sitting in a pew, singing hymns, memorizing Scripture, doodling at her mother's feet as the pastor gave the sermon. After a morning at House Church, where a small group of families, couples, and singles sat in a circle of folding chairs, dressed in a mixture of t-shirts, skirts, and cutoffs, I was very curious to hear her thoughts.

Secretly, I hoped she'd say that *this* was what church was supposed to be: authentic and informal, with lots of personal sharing, some Quaker-like silence, and even a joke or two about our Republican president. I had a sense of pride about the place and was eager to share with others what Christian community *could* be. Instead, she said simply, "It just didn't feel like church to me."

True. House Church is not for everyone. It is unconventional in a number of ways and raises the question of whether it is possible to be a church with no pastor, no building, and no denomination—and with a Statement of Faith and Action that is less than 250 words long.

For the most part, House Church did not emphasize the *words* of its Christian faith. Dad was much the same way. Mom, the daughter of missionaries and a writer-of-sorts, likes words more than Dad did, and admits that this was occasionally a sticking point between them. She wished House Church would work harder at articulating its beliefs. Still, she loves to tell a story about Dad's unspoken faith, and she tells it with a pleased gleam in her eye.

The story takes place at a Learning Center support group meeting. Neither Mom nor Dad had attended this particular gathering, so the story came to them via a friend who had. Apparently, someone at the meeting was in a bit of a huff. "Some people in this group aren't very clear that they are Christian," she said. Even though the speaker didn't use Dad's name, the friend relating the story was certain the speaker was referring to him.

"You should have seen Vivian Headings," the storyteller told my parents, laughing. "She rose straight up in her chair, gathered her breath, and proclaimed, 'Some people *live* their faith!'"

I am grateful to Vivian—for defending Dad, of course, but also for defending the age-old saying that "actions speak louder than words." Believe me, I do think words matter; they sometimes matter very much. But I am grateful to have grown up in a family and a church that understood how creeds and ink-on-paper doctrines can sometimes divide people who might otherwise benefit from engaging one another in conversation. A list of shared beliefs and values can form an important core—a campfire around which a community gathers, but if the list becomes too long, too detailed, too inflexible, our communities become nation-states with boundaries that hold people in and out.[49]

Words can also be hollow when not woven thoughtfully into our everyday lives. This, I think, Dad believed wholeheartedly. Our family's good friend, Dan Charles, puts it this way: "Nelson wasn't much for spiritual and pious words. Sometimes I had the feeling he didn't completely trust them. He certainly wanted to stay far away from anything that might seem like false piety. His was a piety of relationships."[50]

I imagine the questions Dad asked himself most often were not, *Was Jesus really the Son of God, who was born of the virgin Mary, died for my sins, descended into hell, and on the third day resurrected from the dead?* Instead, Dad was asking, *Is my community caring for one another? Are we caring for those in need? And who will fix the broken crate where we store our hymnals, if not I?*

♣

House Church raised me to be a Christian. The adults in the church told me Bible stories in "children's circle" and, when I was thirteen, baptized me at my request. At the time, I believed that Jesus was a great guy, insanely loving, God incarnate. He cared deeply about all the folks the world tended to disregard—the children, the poor, the hungry, the imprisoned. I believed he was a good friend of mine. And I wanted my life to resemble his.

Once I was old enough to have questions about my family's Christian faith, however, I had a pile of them, and I learned very quickly that my parents—and everyone at church—had some of their own. This was a comforting and disturbing realization.

Stories told well, often, and young enough become part of us, like skin. As I grew up, many were added to my story-skin, each influencing my understanding of the world—stories of Anabaptist believers burned at the stake in Europe, of dogs and fire hoses set on blacks in Alabama, of indigenous children swung against walls like baseball bats by Guatemalan paramilitaries, of that man born among straw and manure who lived a life so loving, they killed him at Calvary.

In college, my friends and I tried out new stories and lifestyles—some more experimental than others. We explored passions like French wine, social justice, India, feminism, money—never fully settling into one or another. I have never heard the verb used in this way, but I swear we *talked apart* most things that we had grown up believing. In all our experiments in living and deconstructing our ideologies, we peeled the story-skin from our bodies till we no longer knew what was true.

What I am describing is sometimes called *postmodernism*, an approach to life which defies definitions of truth and reality, and deconstructs foundational ideologies and moralities. In such a world, it is hard to feel at home in any one faith tradition. It is hard to make any truth statements at all without also acknowledging that others' experiences may have taught them differently.

Today, a decade and a half after my Christian baptism at House Church, I still feel at home among Mennonites and people of faith, but I no longer identify strongly as a Christian. You could say that I have spent most of my twenties swimming in the swampy space between *certainty* and *relativism*, both of which are, in my experience, unworkable and unsatisfying. In retrospect, my childhood at Community House Church—while grounded in an explicitly Christian tradition—prepared me somewhat for this postmodern swamp.

"I always thought when I was younger that I would reach forty and suddenly have it all figured out," I remember one church member sharing on a Sunday morning when I was a child. "But any of you young people, take note. That is not at all the case."

On another Sunday, a man's face broke with tears. He was deeply troubled by current events and the Bible's contradictory statements on something—perhaps violence; I no longer remember for sure. He shared his helplessness with the group: "I don't understand sometimes why we don't just throw this book out altogether!"

The honesty and uncertainty of the adults at House Church made a marked impression on me as a child. I learned not to fear questions. I learned to build my life on values instead of rules, and to be slow to judge others. And over the years, I learned to love House Church. The warmth and integrity of its people, along with their compassion, progressive politics, and rejection of dogma, continue to guide me in my own swamp-swimming.

♣

I knew that, over the years, Dad had asked his own share of questions about the traditional teachings of his childhood faith, so when we sat down to talk about the church he and Mom had attended for almost thirty years, I wanted him to tell me about how he balanced the pious places he came from with the less definitive place he found himself now. Had House Church been a raft for him in that in-between swamp?

It was one of our final interviews, and I thought the topic was clear. We would talk a little about Dad's faith journey. Our conversation might venture into his own questions over the years about Christianity and institutional religion. Then we would hunker down into the history-telling of House Church's beginnings up to the present day. Simple.

Instead, we talked about housing cooperatives. That's right. *Co-ops.*

I should not have been surprised that, with Dad's ambivalence around too much "faith talk," we would soon be discussing instead something he had hoped to *do.* We had barely started the conversation when Dad began describing his unrealized hope that he and Mom would some day form a live-in community with other couples, singles, and families from House Church. It seems that, while the Rolling Ridge group worked at developing their intentional community in the woods of West Virginia, Dad was dreaming up an urban version of community, and he hoped that people from the church would help make it happen.

The house we lived in until I was five had no backyard but a wonderful deck that jutted out into the alley. I knew little of the dangers of city alleys or that green, grassy yards existed. This—the wood of our deck and the splash of our two-feet-deep plastic swimming pool—was all I knew, and I was content to run from the laundry room to the pool screaming "On a hot, hot day in July!" (which was the beginning to a song on one of our favorite records) and then splash loudly into the water, with my brother close behind.

"Twenty-seven-twenty," as we called the house with its alley-deck, was located at 2720 Ontario Road. We lived there until I was in kindergarten, December 1985. I didn't understand fully until my conversation with Dad about House Church that the house on Ontario Road was another piece of Dad's vision for what could be.

As he describes in this chapter, he and Mom originally bought the property with a second couple. They co-owned and lived in it together for a number of years, in a smaller version of the larger cooperative Dad hoped would one day be possible.

"I envisioned a group from House Church," he said, "buying a small apartment building and renovating it so each family unit would have its own modest apartment. Other larger spaces could be shared: a library, a shop, and extra guest rooms." The shared mortgage would be more affordable for each individual family. Sharing some living space, lawn equipment, and even childcare would make it possible for everyone in the community to live on a lower income. But, for a number of reasons, this idea never made it very far past Dad's internal drawing board.

Dad and I spoke about many things in the weeks before he died; this was one of the more surprising. I'd had no idea he held onto an unrealized vision that still burned so brightly inside him. He had mentioned this idea, in my memory, only very rarely in the years before his diagnosis, but apparently, it was with him all along. For all of Dad's highly praised "community-building," he seemed to do a lot of his daydreaming quietly and on his own.

House Church meant more to my dad, of course, than a possible springboard into cooperative living. In many ways, the group was his extended family.[51] Dad's six biological brothers have all settled back in Pennsylvania after scattering to other parts of the country and world in their young adult years, many of them living today not far from the farm where they were raised. They understand parts of him better than many of his city friends ever could. Over the years, he bantered with them about football and politics, confided with them about his life, and listened to them share about their own.

But in the city of Washington, I think House Church became Dad's lifeblood, his peers, the nucleus of his wide-reaching support group. When he was diagnosed in January 2005, House Church members were untethered by the news as though they were his brothers, sisters, nieces, and nephews. They helped out in countless ways, provided meal after meal for our family, devotedly read our e-mails, ran errands, sent cards, and visited us in our home.

In addition to these close relationships, House Church provided Dad with another outlet for his gifts, ideas, and explorations in community-building. As part of the budget committee, he gave considerable thought to developing structures for economic sharing. And as a Sunday school teacher (and a dad), he coordinated activities for youth from House Church and other small city churches.

Young people often felt comfortable around my dad, and he became a (first, second, or third) father figure for several teenagers in the church in addition to his own kids' friends. Fourteen-year-old Madeline Dunne stood in tears at an event before Dad's funeral. "I go to House Church, and Nelson was a good friend of mine," she said between breaths. "He was always so nice and always had a smile on his face. I could go to him if I had any problems and needed to talk. . . . He was one of the few adults that I had a lot of respect for."

♣

As to my postmodern swamp-swimming, my ongoing dilemma about naming any truths as truer than others? I don't know that Dad ever resolved all the questions in his box, wrapping it neatly and tying it shut with a ribbon. He left the box open and turned his attention much more toward how to *be* and what to *do* than to clearly articulating his beliefs. He lived his faith.

I made a music-mix CD for Dad and gave it to him for what turned out to be his last Christmas with us. We did not even know he was sick at the time. Later, he told me how grateful he was for one song I had included.

This is my song, Oh God of all the nations,
A song of peace for lands afar and mine.
This is my home, the country where my heart is;
Here are my hopes, my dreams, my sacred shrine.
But other hearts in other lands are beating,
With hopes and dreams as true and high as mine.

"Finlandia," the melody is called.[52] Dad recognized the tune from an old hymn he grew up singing in church. In retrospect, I think this could have been a theme song for Dad's life. His sense of home was so integral to his identity—Ira and Ruth Good's farmhouse, family devotions at breakfast, choir practice at Hammer Creek Mennonite Church.

Even though he left rural Lancaster County for college and then for the city, even though he left the conservative Mennonite church and helped start an ecumenical, relatively progressive house church in D.C., Dad never turned his back on the places, both spiritual and geographical, of his childhood.

This is my home, the country where my heart is;
Here are my hopes, my dreams, my sacred shrine.

Dad tried to stand on a bridge between his traditional Mennonite roots and his more pluralistic life. Mom tells me that in his twenties he continued to attend his home church, Hammer Creek Mennonite, on Sunday mornings even while taking apart the faith of his childhood in philosophy classes he was taking at Millersville State Teachers College.[53]

But other hearts in other lands are beating,
With hopes and dreams as true and high as mine.

This seems to me the magic bridge over the swamp. It requires an ability to stand solidly on my own two feet, firmly planted in my roots and my core commitments (which include: loving as best I can, seeking justice for all people, and sitting with an ever-expansive sense of Mystery) while still opening my hands to others different from me, and to their "hopes and dreams as true and high as mine." This is not an answer but a North Star. I believe Dad strove toward it, imperfectly and with humility. Yes, humility. That may be most important of all.

Father's Voice
A Place of Belonging

Community House Church, in many ways, has fit my idea of what I want in a faith community. As Betty and I visited churches after our two years on W Street, I was not looking for a traditional church. I had questions about institutionalized religion as codifying the ways that one enters the kingdom of Heaven. I felt that a church that started instead at the level of community—of listening and sharing openly with one another—provided a better opportunity for discovering who God is and for exploring the relevance of the New Testament in today's society and times. I wanted a church with flexibility, openness, and room for searching. I was also looking for a church group that was interested in trying creative community structures—different ways of being church beyond simply getting together for worship on Sunday mornings.

My telling of the House Church story really begins with several strands of vision that I hoped to weave together in my life: cooperative housing, shared resources, and authentic community-building. Only pieces of this vision have been realized in the church community, but in those pieces, I have found a home.

__Our Church Hunt__

When we were living at Friendship Flat, Betty and I attended Peabody Street Mennonite Church for two years. The church was a very conservative expression of faith stemming from Lancaster Conference, an organization of Mennonite churches in Pennsylvania. At Peabody Street, people tended to dress in plain suits and coverings. We didn't feel particularly comfortable there, but we attended nonetheless as a way of supporting Lancaster Conference, which sponsored our voluntary service unit.

After finishing with voluntary service in 1972, we began attending Church of the Saviour at 2025 Massachusetts Avenue. This was an ecumenical and dynamic church, very committed to "inward" spiritual development *and* "outward" work in the world. Members of the church were deeply involved in the city's social concerns through their "mission groups." It was a good place for us at the time.[54]

Meanwhile, a different group of families and individuals had begun gathering in homes once a week for supper.[55] Eventually, the group started to meet on Sunday evenings, followed by a worship service. Several other families joined them, and Betty and I visited several times.

We wanted to settle somewhere. In the end, we chose House Church in part because its core values seemed akin to our Anabaptist-Mennonite beliefs and values, even though the church has never declared itself Mennonite. Betty and I were also drawn to House Church because of the children. Betty was pregnant with Ryan at the time. A number of couples in the church already had children. The presence of families made it attractive to us.

And, as I will describe later, I was looking for a group that might do some creative thinking around a community housing effort. I was looking for a group that might consider living together and sharing resources. The small and dynamic nature of House Church, with its emphasis on lifestyle concerns and

Christian faith, seemed like it could be the birthplace of a co-operative housing project.

Betty and I became members soon after Ryan was born in 1978. We have attended what is now called Community House Church ever since.

__*Making Changes*__

During the 1980s, we continued to meet in homes for worship and a shared meal every Sunday. We were getting smaller as some of our group left, and we weren't drawing many new members, partly because people couldn't find where we were meeting. Sometime in the mid-1980s, we began to feel stretched by the high levels of participation the church required from all of us. We questioned whether we could continue to exist, but we weren't ready to give the church up altogether.

We made several changes. For one thing, we decided to meet only three Sunday mornings a month for worship, which took less of our energy and allowed us to visit more established congregations if we wanted. We continued to be a lay fellowship, without a pastor, but for a few years, we paid members to be worship coordinators. Even after we stopped paying, we kept the worship-coordinator model, taking turns in the position, so that our Sunday morning worships were better planned.

We also tried to create more consistency in where we met, rotating among three houses.[56] By the 1990s, we were getting too big to meet in homes and began renting space at Catholic University as our regular place of worship, which made it even easier for people to find us. Our attendance grew substantially, with up to fifty or sixty people attending on Sundays. We have kept the name "House Church" even though we never again met regularly in homes.

Even as we have become more structured in our worship planning and meeting places, House Church still strongly emphasizes participation from everyone. It is not a leader-focused church. Anyone who attends is invited to participate in all parts of the worship, in small groups, and on retreats.

__No Building. No Pastor. No Denomination.__

House Church has done a number of things differently than most churches. Even after outgrowing living rooms, we have always rented space, never owning our own facility. All we need is a room. We set up chairs in a circle, bring our own hymnals and decorations, and at the end of the service, clean up and leave the room as we found it.

Every ten years or so, we have reviewed the question of whether to buy a church building, but as long as we could find alternatives that were much more cost-effective, we have preferred not to. We haven't wanted a large portion of our budget to be tied up in owning and maintaining our own property. When you own a building, it not only absorbs a lot of funds. It requires time and management to care for it. It also tends to be inefficient in that the church only needs the facility for a limited amount of time every week. We have chosen instead to use facilities that are primarily used for other services during the week: a university lounge or classroom, a housing organization, and a neighborhood-services center.

We have also faced the question of having a pastor. I'm not sure we were ever in a position to have a pastor, because we didn't have the amount of money needed to support one, so the decision was dictated partly by economics. But we are also strongly attracted to having a lay fellowship. It encourages many people to participate in creating worship life and planning community activities, developing a broad base of leadership. We've never had much debate over who is in charge, because everybody has to lead different pieces. Nobody has enough time to provide all of the leadership.

Each month, a different person acts as the worship coordinator, planning services on a given theme. Every Sunday, a different person gives what we call the "meditation," which fills the role a sermon plays in most churches. Others take turns leading music, telling the children's story, reading Scripture, and teaching Sunday school.

We also have small groups that usually meet twice a month, a members' group that meets once a month, and committees that coordinate different aspects of church life. There are retreats—at Rolling Ridge and elsewhere—and various informal activities that help build community life.

Once a year, everyone is invited to a unique gathering we call our "cutting edges retreat." At the retreat we ask, *What are our spiritual cutting edges, individually and communally? What are the things keeping us awake at night—the areas where we need the most support from the church and want to hear others' thoughts and feelings?* Through this process, we plan the themes we want our worship services to address in the coming year. At a deeper level, though, we are re-assessing, every year, what our core values and beliefs are as a community, adapting them as our spiritual and social needs change.

So the House Church community is based on much more than a preacher, a church building, and a Sunday morning service. Small group life, retreats, and members' meetings are just as important for our identity as the Sunday service itself. I think one of the church's greatest strengths is its many opportunities for participation. You really can't attend on an ongoing basis without getting drawn into contributing in some way. The participatory nature of the church results in diversified leadership, so that no one person's personality shapes the life of the community.

♣

And why are we an independent faith community, unaffiliated with a larger church denomination? In the church's original supper group, a number of the families and individuals had participated in the ecumenical Church of the Saviour. They were influenced by its clear effort to not become a part of denominationalism, which it saw as a weakness that kept Christians apart.

If we were to explore belonging to a denomination, there was also the obvious question of which we would belong to. House Church folks have come from a variety of Anabaptist and other denominational groups. Joining the Mennonite church would seem the most likely, but belonging to a denomination with an unwelcoming stance toward gays and lesbians has been unacceptable for many in our group. Generally, many of the people who have joined House Church over the years have been attracted to the church because of the fact that it isn't burdened down by the requirements of a denomination.

As a congregation unaffiliated with a denomination, however, there is a risk that House Church will not have sources of accountability. We do have a network of relationships with other small churches that, I think, serve the same purpose—groups we are connected to through Rolling Ridge and personal relationships. In many ways, our sense of accountability to our commitments—like caring for one another, the environment, and greater social justice—is achieved through these networks. This is a different kind of accountability. In contrast to the top-down accountability of denominations, ours is more of a conversation among equals.

__A Vision for Cooperative Housing__

Over the years, many have been drawn to House Church because of its strong community life. From the beginning, however, I have always wanted something more. I imagined extensive systems of shared economics, more shared activities, and collaborative housing projects.

As a young adult, I was developing an overall vision for enhancing community life through cooperative living arrangements. During the late 1960s and early 1970s, many in my generation shared a general interest in community. Groups throughout the country were developing "common pot" community houses, in which everybody combined their incomes, lived together, and ate together, thereby reducing their everyday living costs.

In general, these households didn't last very long, sometimes because people were crowded together too tightly, or because the larger group setting proved difficult when children became involved.

My interest was not in developing an intentional community with a common pot. I believed that in the long term, this might not be sustainable. I hoped instead to develop other means of sharing resources that allowed families more autonomy. I envisioned a group of couples and families from House Church buying and renovating a small apartment building so each family unit would have its own modest apartment, while other larger spaces could be shared. By living in the same building, or in houses close together, we could share more resources (whether laundry machines, heat expenses, or garden tools) and, as a result, Lve comfortably on lower incomes.

I was continually exploring ways to make this happen. When Betty and I bought our first house at 2720 Ontario Road in Adams Morgan, we co-owned the property with another couple, Herb and Ginny Buckwalter. I hoped that this could be a first step toward exploring ways of doing cooperative housing. The house was larger than we needed for one family, which allowed us to create an upstairs unit and a downstairs unit, with a large living room at the front of the house that we shared. We also had a small apartment in the back of the house, which we rented to a single person.

In my mind, this was only a step toward a larger vision that involved more families and greater shared ownership, but several factors made it difficult to take this vision further: rising housing prices, zoning issues, and the challenge of finding families who wanted to explore this with us *at the same time.*

When Herb and Ginny moved to Canada in 1977, we bought their half of 2720 Ontario Road and began looking for a family to replace them in the upstairs unit of the house. Shortly, David and Sharon Lloyd moved in and rented from us. We didn't sell any shares to David and Sharon, in part because housing prices were going up so fast that if they stayed only a few years and then left, we would have had to buy their half back at a much higher price. The Lloyds also were not ready to jump into a housing commitment at that level.

Later, when our family was looking to leave Ontario Road, I was ambivalent about moving to the row house on Kenyon Street where we now live because I still wished I could somehow find a way to do a cooperative housing project. But I was discovering that finding the right property would be almost impossible. Only certain areas are zoned correctly for multiple family housing, and we wanted a neighborhood that would be multicultural, multi-racial, *and* affordable. Many appealing neighborhoods in D.C. were getting quite expensive, and we knew that we—and the families who might potentially join us in a cooperative housing arrangement—would not be able to afford the shared mortgage.

There was also the problem of mismatched timing with other families. To pull off such a project, we would have needed to find enough families who were all at the right stage of life, with enough energy to get it going. I remember Marlin and Barb Good,[57] for example, were seriously exploring the possibility of creating a housing co-op in the 1990s. I had a lot of interest in working with them and felt I had a lot of experience in navigating housing issues and developing initiatives, but it was the wrong time for me. I was deeply involved in my work with the Thurgood Marshall Center[58] and felt I couldn't put time and energy into something new. By the time I was finished with the Center, Marlin and Barb had left D.C. altogether.

I expect also that my vision for a collaborative housing effort—specifically with members of House Church—never came to be partly because of my own unwillingness to give up my autonomy as a person, to give leadership to making it happen. It also seemed to me that new people joining House Church viewed it more as a Sunday morning church option than we had in the early days. The group's primary identity had shifted somewhat from "community" to "church." I had trouble creating any momentum behind my vision.

Even though Betty and I never became part of an intentional live-in community with House Church, we have found ways to use our home as a place for building community with the church and others. At different points over the years, the Learning Center support group, the Rolling Ridge group, and House Church have all met in our living room.

Our current house also has two small apartments. While these apartments are completely separated from our living space, they have provided good neighborly relationships for us and for our children, as well as providing added security. We figured our children were safer coming home from school if one of our tenants was home, and our house was always less likely to be broken into because of the number of people coming and going from the property. Rent payments also helped diversify our sources of income as a family.

__A Middle Ground__

While House Church never became the communal effort I had once envisioned, it did embody many of the same ideals. Perhaps what we developed in House Church—through structures that allowed for sharing resources—has been a healthy middle ground.

I led the way on a few of these structures for shared economics. For one thing, I negotiated with a Mennonite agency called Mennonite Mutual Aid (MMA) in the 1970s to take us on as one of its member groups, given our strong Anabaptist identity. We have been members of MMA ever since, which has provided matching funds for couples going through adoption processes, for medical needs, and sometimes for basic living costs. It has also provided a medical insurance option for individuals or families that belong to House Church. The connection to the mutual aid agency has become a real benefit.

We also provide small scholarships for our college students and have our own mutual fund, internal to the church, which provides grants and short-term loans for people in the congregation with special financial needs. We have helped students through school and families through job transitions and housing difficulties. It was crucial to me to set up the structures that allow us to help each other out in this way.

In House Church, we also share resources beyond money. When a family is facing a significant transition—a birth, a car accident, or illness—the rest of us provide meals for them. And, as I've talked about already, we share the Rolling Ridge Retreat House with other local congregations and groups. As a "partner group" of Rolling Ridge, we have access to the Retreat House for weekend retreat experiences, including retreats for Sunday school classes.

__Clarifying Our Identity__

The fact that House Church is non-denominational and encourages lay participation has certainly *not* left us conflict-free. Over the years a number of issues have surfaced and sometimes resurfaced, creating notable markers in our development as a congregation.

Mission

One such marker came just as Betty and I were joining House Church. Jim and Grace Dickerson were discussing with the group their desire to be part of a mission-based church. They felt called to start an interracial church that could be a worshipping community for inner-city families.

Others in House Church believed this was a great ministry but not one they felt called to. A church that focused too much on *outward mission*, and even on *inward spirituality*, they said, neglected to create a sustainable community that would support families.[59]

One of the early members of House Church, as I recall, had grown up in a pastor's family, very focused on serving others, and was now much more interested in being a church that served the people who attended it. I, too, felt that focusing too much on mission could mean neglecting community.

While we supported Jim and Grace in their desire for an interracial, mission-oriented church, it was becoming clear that House Church was taking on a different emphasis. These differences caused considerable tension and finally, Jim and Grace decided to leave.[60]

Doctrines and Stances

Several years later, in the 1980s, Terry and Tammy Colvin also decided to leave House Church. They were interested in a church with more clarity of beliefs and a more charismatic expression of faith, whereas our worship was lowkey, and our shared beliefs were somewhat ambiguous.

It was becoming clear that House Church did not consider dogma crucial and focused instead on personal sharing. That value has been sustained in the church over the years. The commitment statement we eventually composed, our Statement of Faith and Action, focuses on faith as action, rather than on statements of belief.

Nobody has to fit a particular position or say a particular creed to be part of the group. One can be completely unsure of what he or she believes and still belong to House Church. I personally have struggled with the question of doctrines, wondering if we should make more absolute statements of belief. On one hand, I think we do need to focus on what it is that draws us together as a body of believers. On the other hand, there is a great benefit to not creating boundaries, and acknowledging that a church is a community of members in flux, each of us on our own changing journey of faith.

Over the years, we have sometimes talked about identify-
ing our core values in more concrete ways—peace and justice,
grace, and community, among others. I think it is this core that
defines House Church, not a long list of doctrinal positions. As
I remember it, House Church's distaste for dogma, and our
openness to people who are searching, was becoming clearer to
the group about the time that Terry and Tammy left the
church. In the years since, some have left over this issue, while
others have been drawn to House Church because of it.

I remember the issue of infant baptism surfacing sometime
in the 1980s. House Church certainly had Anabaptist leanings,
but we had not made a point of taking a stance against baptiz-
ing infants. On several occasions, parents in the fellowship who
came out of church backgrounds that practiced infant baptism
wished to have their children baptized at the church as infants—and the issue became a lightning rod.

Some at members' meeting felt it would be unacceptable
for us to practice infant baptism, because they came from a heritage in which sixteenth-century Anabaptists died for the belief
that baptism should mark an *adult's* decision of faith. We discussed the issue at length and, in the end, agreed to support the
parents by having the baptism in the church. The difference of
opinion became a grace, because it brought to light one value
dear to the church: to be inclusive and not to draw lines.

There has also been some discussion around abortion.
Shouldn't we take a position, some asked, that was more clearly
pro-choice? Others in the church said, "No, no. House Church
cannot take that position; that isn't where we are." So those
who wanted to participate in pro-choice marches did, but we
didn't make it an official stance of the church.

And should we take an outspoken position on the gay
issue? As we have discussed this question, it is very clear that we
want to be a welcoming fellowship (we have had gay members),
but there is also caution about being too positional or making
an issue of it by speaking out in the larger Christian church.

Size

At times in House Church's history, as the number of people in our congregation has risen and fallen, our size has been a point of discussion.

In the mid-1990s, there were more people than ever before showing up at our weekly members' meetings. This changed the chemistry of our decision-making. As a group of fifteen, there was a lot more space for informal sharing when we worked through issues. When our group grew to thirty to thirty-five, we worried that the discernment process would have to be formalized. We even discussed creating a group of elders.[61] We also discussed redefining membership, which was a controversial idea.

About this same time, several things happened that changed the size of the church. One or two couples put out a call for others to join them in creating a Sunday evening church. They wanted a small home church, somewhat like House Church had been in its early years, with more informal sharing instead of a programmed worship service. This second fellowship—known as Evening Church—formed with strong support from and mutuality with House Church. A number of families and individuals have chosen to attend Evening Church instead of or in addition to House Church's morning service.

On top of that, several families moved away from Washington, further reducing our size. Some went overseas to do development work. Some moved back to rural areas where they had grown up. So the issues created by our increasing size seemed to dissolve without any significant changes in structure or definitions of membership.

Though the conflicts over mission, doctrine, baptism, and church size have been difficult and have sometimes resulted in important people leaving, it is through these conversations over the years that House Church has developed more clarity about its identity.

__What We Can and Can't Do__

There's a unique and subtle ethos about House Church that member John Swarr has held up all these many years. He emphasizes that as a church we carry out our mission together to the extent that we have the capacity to do so. We don't bring a lot of "should's" and "have-to's." If we don't have the energy and the lay capacity to achieve something, then we don't necessarily do it.

As a result, there are many things we probably don't do as well as a large, well-staffed church could. Right now, House Church is being tested in relation to my illness and coming death. We have pulled together in remarkable ways, but I have had to face the fact that House Church has no pastor to provide a dying person with pastoral support. So I, who have advocated for the lay model, have decided to reach out to a pastor from another church. In doing so, I feel like I am acknowledging that we are not able to provide everything. We also haven't done very well in relation to baptism, teaching, marriage counseling, and other services a pastor is trained to provide.

When initiatives take off in House Church, it requires that somebody feel called to it and that there be a shared vision to sustain it. At points, that has kept us from trying to do too much. In many ways, it's amazing that we continue to survive after all these years. I credit our survival in part to this ethos: "We'll do just what we can do, and what we can't do, we don't do." We focus on doing what we think is really important.

__Coming Home__

Betty and I have had fairly unique roles in House Church, particularly recently. We have been part of the congregation longer than most and have been the oldest members of the congregation for a number of years. There are times I have wished for "peers," I suppose, but I don't think about it much. There are a number of people at House Church that I consider peers, even if they are younger than I am.

I never became a formal leader at House Church. I was moderator of the members' group, perhaps our most defined leadership role, for just one year. But I have never played a strong role in worship planning. I have taught Sunday school for middle-school and high-school youth and helped coordinate with other youth groups in small city churches. And I've done considerable work on the budget and facilities committees.

Even though I have very rarely had any formal leadership roles at House Church, I have been subtly aware of what might be called an informal deference to me as a leader—likely because of my age, my length of time in the group, maybe my personality, and my experiences working with informal organizations. In general, House Church is consensus-oriented, but the danger with informal power structures like ours is that some members of a group unofficially develop more influence. I have felt sometimes that my opinions are noticed while others' are less likely to be heard. I don't think I have overused my power—I certainly hope not.

I don't think Community House Church is made for everyone, but for me, it has been a real inspiration to be part of a community that has so welcomed my gifts and been open to finding new ways of being church to one another. And even though House Church never became a communal church to the extent I had originally hoped for, it has provided a place where families and individuals can find others who are asking similar questions—a place where questions are acceptable, as well as beliefs.

I think of House Church as a place of belonging. It has been important to me in helping me feel at home here in the city. Rather than just having a scattering of friends, I have an extended family of sorts. It is a place I have felt loved, where I have been able to love and include others, to experience other people's gifts and offer my own. In that sense, House Church has been for me a coming home.

june 4, 2005

Two weeks ago, we celebrated Dad's sixty-first birthday, and Father's Day will be here in another two. I have puzzled over how to celebrate. Dad was always hard to shop for, but this year, material gifts seem all but ridiculous. What would he do with a new drill?

Mostly, I want Dad to know that my love for him is bigger than the woods—I don't know how one body can hold it all. Over the years, his abounding enthusiasm about me has again and again bolstered my shaky self-confidence, teaching me to be deeply comfortable with myself—a priceless gift.

If my grief is as big as my love, it will rip me up, and today, the prospect frightens me.

I look out the back window and remember the countless basketball games we've played in the alley. Ryan would guard Jason, and I would take Dad with his left-handed hook shot, practically unstoppable and famous among our friends. Dad and Ryan built the backboard from old floorboards, and it has hung off the back of Mom and Dad's garage for years. I catch myself. It's going to be a long time before I feel comfortable calling it "Mom's garage." Mom and Dad just go together like Philadelphia and Eagles. How can one be possible without the other?

I think I must accept that this is going to be hard and depression may be a gentle—if unwanted—companion. Getting angry at my sadness will not make it go away. I pray the memories hold more richness than the present which, to me, seems washed in a terrible fog.

Life has slowed down considerably. There are no more doctors' appointments, no more radiation, no more chemotherapy. I am working less and spending more time at home. I am grateful for the little routine I have: Every night, those of us who are home gather in a circle. We read cards and e-mails, which continue to arrive almost daily. We remember and share about the day's highlights and hardships. And we read aloud from the Psalms or a Celtic book of prayers. Dad values this time deeply, and I have come to feel the same.

Dad and I are close to finishing the interviews. I am transcribing and editing the ones we have already done, so Dad
can read them. If he is too tired, as he often is, I read them to
him and he suggests changes. I am so grateful for all the time
with him—to be working together on one last project.

Mostly, though, these are days for being, not doing. A
friend recently shared with me her reflections on midwifery,
how being present to women in labor is much like accompanying the dying. Like midwives, we keep Dad company, do
our best to comfort him and ease his pain, and, ultimately,
wait for the body to take over.

Dying, it seems, is a lot like childbirth. The baby in utero
has no idea what's on the other side of that birth canal; she's
been in the dark, breathing water as long as she can remember. I have heard that in some ancient cultures, those who attended births were often the same people who cared for the
dying. I like this sense of purpose and identity: for the time
being, I am a midwife to my father.

This past weekend, Mom, Dad, Jason, and I drove to
Lancaster, Pennsylvania, to the farm where Dad used to get
up early every morning to milk the cows before school (a fact
he repeated often for his late-rising children). This is the place
where he was born and raised—a large white farmhouse with
painted shutters, barn and silo, swings overlooking the
stream.

At Dad's request, we spent the afternoon in the living
room with Dad's six brothers and their wives. The day's
agenda was storytelling. They told of childhood games and
mischief, illness, near disasters, and visits to the grandparents'. Their stories, laughter, and even some apologies filled
the room. Jason and I felt almost like privileged guests, wit-
nesses to something final, and therefore, sacred.

Back at home, we have begun talking about the logistics:
viewing, cremation, burial. When we do, I find myself being
difficult, and crying on the couch.

I have an impossible time putting the feeling into words,
but it is stronger than I would have thought. I do not want to
see the body. Not after the funeral home has dressed it up,
made it up, and injected it with formaldehyde. I have been at

two open-casket funerals this spring, and now, when I think of the deceased, my mind too readily recalls the coffins—their faces cold, powdered, not quite themselves—when what I most want to remember are their living, breathing personalities.

And soon it will be Dad's turn. He is part of the conversation, which makes it all the more unbearable. Ultimately, he wants to be cremated and interred next to Mom. They have already decided where. Mom feels strongly that there should be a viewing, that some people need to see the body before they can truly grieve the loss.

In the end, we compromise. Dad's body will be available for viewing in a side room, but none of us will stand beside it in a greeting line. If I choose not to see his body lying in a coffin, I won't have to. After the funeral, it will be cremated and given to us in a wooden box.

The conversation makes me ache inside and out. I am glad when it is over.

We also talk about the funeral events and decide that we would like to have sandwiches, fruit, and drinks afterward for everyone who attends. Friends from House Church will coordinate the food, and we, as a family, will plan much of the funeral service ourselves, after Dad is gone.

At some point in the conversation, Dad looks around at us with a twinkle in his eye. "Man," he says, "I'm sure going to miss that sandwich bar."

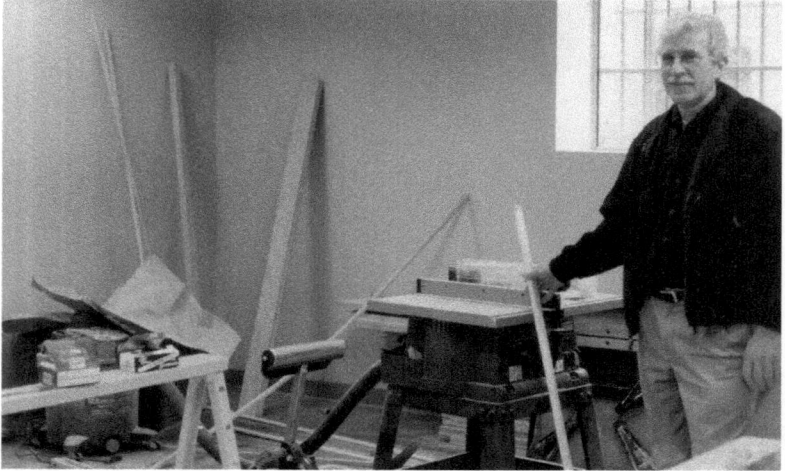

Nelson was involved for nearly fourteen years in the restoration of the historic 12th Street YMCA building in D.C.'s Shaw neighborhood.
Photo credit: Deborah Good, future site of the Learning Center in the Thurgood Marshall building, 2000

Chapter 6

THURGOOD MARSHALL CENTER

Daughter's Voice
Color Lines

I had a history teacher in high school who believed all white people were racists. I remember slinking into my seat, feeling small and pale, fighting the idea that my white skin could stain my whole being, making me bad, through and through.

Sitting on the stairs at home after one of the first days of the school year, I discussed the situation with Dad. I was angry, hard as the wood beneath my tailbone. He was understanding, but he did not coddle me.

"I can understand her assertion that white people are racists."

"What do you mean? There's nothing we can do about our skin color!" Honestly, I was probably on the edge of tears. In my mind, I was on the receiving end of more racism from peers (*What you think you're doing, white girl?*) than I ever gave out. "How can I possibly be racist just because of how I look?"

"There is a difference between personal racism and institutional racism," Dad explained, slowly. "I think Ms. Green is

probably talking about institutional or structural racism. Many
of this country's power and financial structures benefit whites,
which in turn benefits you." Dad liked to leave long pauses between his sentences. I was never sure if he simply wanted us to
hear every word he said, or if his brain actually moved a little
more slowly—more intentionally—than most.

"Not only that, but Europe and white America have privileged themselves for several centuries, so even though you
didn't ask for it, you were born into it. It's like we inherited centuries of privilege, giving us a disproportionate amount of
power and influence in many situations. I suppose one could
argue that this makes us racists."

I wasn't convinced, but if anyone was listening closely, they
could probably hear the creaking of my widening racial consciousness.

Ah, *race*. My dad's stories so far have been peppered with
the theme, but in a book set mostly in Washington, D.C.,
there's no way I'm getting away with just pepper. The mostly
African-American city practically floats on its racial undercur-
rents. And though legal segregation was outlawed nearly half a
century ago, the District—and much of this country—are still
largely segregated along color lines.

♣

In 1988, Dad was hired to help with a project whose primary swell of energy and purpose rose out of the African-American community. The goal was to save a historic building in
Washington's Shaw neighborhood from the ever-hungry hands
of developers and restore it as a center for community use. As
with many of his involvements, Dad had no way of knowing, at
the outset, that his commitment to the work would entangle
him for over a decade. The newly renovated Thurgood Marshall
Center for Service and Heritage opened its doors in April 2000,
and by the time of Dad's farewell party the following year, he
had been involved with the project for nearly fourteen years.

The historic building in question, the first full-service black YMCA in the country, is located near 12th and U Streets in northwest Washington, a short walk from the block of W Street where my parents spent their first two years in the city.

During much of the twentieth century, the YMCA thrived, serving as an important neighborhood hub and a haven for black young people. They played basketball in the gym, took photography classes from neighborhood volunteers, and developed a sense of responsibility and leadership. Over time, however, the building fell into disrepair and financial trouble, and in 1982, the historic landmark closed its doors and sat abandoned, a target for developers who would likely convert it into profitable condominiums.

In 1987, FLOC[62] and the Shaw Heritage Trust, a newly formed neighborhood organization, partnered in the effort to purchase and renovate the building. Dad was hired to help with fundraising and coordinating the restoration, though it is hard to describe in so few words exactly what his job entailed.

As a child, I hated when people asked me what my father did for a living, because there was no easy teacher-doctor-sales-clerk answer. He wrote a lot of documents. He went to meetings. He spoke on the phone with lawyers and architects, board members and builders. When my brothers and I complained enough about Dad's lack of job title, he finally concocted one as an answer for everyone who asked us. "He's a project coordinator," we'd say. Unfortunately, this mostly led to raised eyebrows and further questioning, so I usually managed a few lines about "the first black YMCA" and "restoration project" and "working with several nonprofits."

In reality, his was a multi-faceted job. When Dad was leaving the project—or, better said, when the renovation was completed and Dad's job phased out—a board member who couldn't make it to his farewell party sent him a letter. *The Thurgood Marshall Center is the result of the work of many, many people*, she wrote, *but you are the one who day in and day out, has held things together and kept [them] on track even in the face of setbacks, doubts, and disappointments.* And there were plenty of setbacks: lightning that struck the chimney not once but twice, funds that fell through unexpectedly, a stench in the women's restroom that turned out to be a plumbing problem.

You have had to become, she went on, *a Jack-of-all trades: financial management, building design and construction, negotiation, building management, event coordination, and even janitorial services! And you have done all these willingly, never saying, "That's not my job." Quite a record!*[63]

♣

Restoring the historic YMCA building involved a collaboration that was noteworthy in many ways, and I am proud of Dad's involvement in it. For many of my growing up years, the project was Dad's primary work (hence my dilemmas around describing it for questioners). Still, of all his involvements, it is the one I know the least about and the one I feel least connected to. This was, in part, because of Dad's ambiguous job description. But I suspect there was a larger reason we never put words to—larger in the sense of societal, unconscious, and ever-present. Larger in the sense of *racial.*

I was born and raised in a city that is well over fifty percent black. I attended a bilingual elementary school where more than a quarter of my classmates spoke Spanish at home, many of them recent immigrants from U.S.-backed, war-wracked El Salvador. Today, I live on a block of mostly African-American families in West Philadelphia.

I just wrote an impressive graduate application essay on my "multicultural" upbringing and surroundings. My essay, however, omitted one of the most shameful confessions of my life thus far: Despite the diversity of my schools and neighborhoods, despite my hefty in-and-out-of-school education in antiracism, black history, multicultural awareness, and progressive politics, despite my great desire that it be otherwise—the vast majority of people I consider confidants, collaborators, and friends could trace their dominant ancestral lines to Europe.

There is no doubt we live in a racially divided country. I am amazed how even an interracial effort like the Thurgood Marshall project, organized by well-meaning, liberal folks committed to preserving a piece of D.C.'s rich African-American history, could not break the color lines in my dad's life in the ways I would have imagined. I rarely met anyone from his work at the Thurgood Marshall Center. I never played with their African-American children. As far as I know, Dad never spent time in their homes or at their cookouts.

Work was work, and Dad worked hard. But at the end of the day, Dad packed up his briefcase and came home to us, his white-skinned family. The communities that composed his life—at House Church and Rolling Ridge—were almost entirely white. Much of the segregation in our lives, I realize, has as much to do with class as with race, but class was not the issue here: the men and women Dad worked with at the Thurgood Marshall Center were, like our family, middle class and well-educated. Still, Dad never tried to integrate his racially diverse work world with his homogeneous personal life. Most of the people I know are equally imperfect.

The reasons for this racial divide in my dad's life and in my own are multi-layered and highly sensitive, a tapestry woven tightly with culture, history, violence, and a grossly unequal distribution of resources. I will not attempt a full explanation in these few paragraphs, but I will say that I am endlessly frustrated and disappointed. The depth of separation between the races persists long past desegregation and reaches into the most progressive of circles.

This is not about *just getting along* or seeing past color to where we can meet each other as equals. Talking only about personal racism does not even begin to touch the depths—indeed, the entire oceans—of economic and power structures in this country that seem to cycle tirelessly in favor of lighter skin. And yet I would argue that, on another level, it *is* about *just getting along*, about just talking frankly with each other over fish and chips, over coffee or beer, visiting each other in our homes, introducing our children.

Even when we can get there in our heads, when and how will we ever break the lines in our own social lives and our organizing? We have a long way to go.

♣

At Dad's farewell party from the Thurgood Marshall Center, he was given a plaque recognizing his "extraordinary commitment and conscientious service" and his "long-lasting and exemplary devotion to the Thurgood Marshall Center." People who had worked with him over the past fourteen years stood and offered words of praise and acclamation. Thomasina Yearwood, the Center's first executive director and an African-American woman, thanked Dad for believing in her abilities as a leader. Jerry Levine, a Jewish lawyer whose firm had done considerable pro bono work for the project, described Dad as a *mensch*, a Yiddish word reserved for the most upright and honorable of people.

Then our family's good friend, Jim Dickerson, explained why Dad was squirming under all the praise. "I can tell you that what is happening right now is one of the hardest things Nelson has ever done," he said. The spotlight was never Dad's favorite place to be.[64]

This willingness to generally avoid center-stage was exactly what made Dad—imperfections aside—quite well-suited for an interracial setting like the Thurgood Marshall Center. He was unusually content to listen to the hopes and directions of others and to work mostly in the background. As Mom puts it, he rarely, if ever, tooted his own horn. I imagine that a different white man, one looking for prestige or accolades, would have created considerable tension in such a setting. Dad believed in the significance of the project—for FLOC, for the Shaw neighborhood, and for African-Americans everywhere. Is it too altruistic to suggest that Dad's commitment to celebrating and preserving African-American heritage was enough to drive his work?

Heritage was a word Dad understood. When I came home from school as a child, frustrated that I could not be black and therefore proud of my heritage—it was, after all, people of European descent who had enslaved, raped, and subjugated the world over the past few centuries—my parents would remind me that I, like my African-American classmates, did have a heritage I could be proud of. I was a Mennonite, they said. I came from a line of simple and faithful people, a line which stretched from the peaceful farmers of Lancaster County all the way back to the radical Anabaptists who died for their faith in sixteenth-century Europe.

Dad's identity was well-rooted in this Mennonite soil, and I expect his love and respect for his own heritage drew him to his work at the Thurgood Marshall Center. While Dad shared a love of culture and heritage with the African-Americans involved in the project, however, he admits that he did not tune into a significant cultural difference that would ultimately complicate the project's success. As Dad describes later in this chapter, he brought to his work a "more with less" approach to running organizations, an approach he carried in his invisible knapsack along with the other values and practices of his Mennonite background.

More with less meant running an organization on a modest-to-low budget. It meant cleaning one's own office instead of hiring a cleaning service. It meant that Dad sometimes took the lawnmower from our basement to cut the grass at the Thurgood Marshall Center instead of paying someone else to do it. In contrast, others at the Center considered it more important that this historic landmark maintain a polished and professional appearance, with hired cleaning and support services.

It is ironic that the values of Dad's own ethnic heritage would clash with those of the African-Americans who would manage the Thurgood Marshall Center long after his job was done. This clash had unforeseen consequences.

When Dad wrote the budget for the building shortly before he left, he assumed that the organizational culture of the Thurgood Marshall Center would mimic his own more-with-less variety. Like all assumptions, Dad wore this one like clothing, largely unaware of it, and he probably never articulated it clearly to the others in the organization. As a result, he significantly under-budgeted what the Thurgood Marshall Center would spend in maintaining the building over the next five years. The Center was forced to raise the rent for its tenants, a shift that Dad thinks contributed to FLOC's financial crises and eventual move from the building.

♣

Dad did not talk about his work much around the supper table at home, but I do remember visiting the building with him a few times. Before the renovations, he walked me and my brothers through the basement with its empty, neglected swimming pool, and up the dirty, creaking staircase. Over Thanksgiving weekend several years later, our family returned to the Twelfth Street building, five months before it opened. The basement swimming pool had been replaced with the carpeted hallways of the FLOC Learning Center. The historic staircase had been restored and the railings polished. A sign over the side entrance read, "Thurgood Marshall Center," in sharp, gold letters. I remember Dad's quiet pride, his sense of satisfaction at a job well done.

By the time of our interview in spring 2005, however, the Thurgood Marshall Center was in transition. FLOC had plans to downsize and move out of the building. Dad expressed disappointment that his original plans for the building's use did not prove sustainable, but he remained hopeful "that other groups might replace FLOC, and that the Thurgood Marshall Center will continue to serve the community in decades to come."

Our family has lost all ties to the Thurgood Marshall Center, a fact that sits right alongside the racial divides that always kept us separated from Dad's work there. It saddens me. I recently stopped by the building for the first time in several years. It may have been a personal effort to scratch the surface of that sadness. I was also hoping, I think, to find a little of my dad in the polished wooden floors and historic staircase climbing upward.

I stood in the space Dad had helped make possible and felt both foreign and grateful. It was obvious that, even with FLOC and the Learning Center no longer there, the Thurgood Marshall Center for Service and Heritage was still standing as a classy and historic landmark and operating as a hub for the African-American community.

Two years earlier, at Dad's memorial service, two well-dressed African-American men emerged from the sea of mostly white faces to pay their respects to my mom. Norris Dodson and Charles Countee were key players in the Thurgood Marshall project; they had learned of the funeral from the newspaper.

Near the entrance to the church where the memorial service was held, we had arranged large white pages on a table, for notes and signatures. Later, after the pages were bound together into a guest book, I read through them and found this:

To the Good family—
Nelson was the rock of our development of the Thurgood Marshall Center, and I shall always be grateful that you allowed us to borrow him for such a long time. Without his tireless effort and dedicated work, we would not have saved and redeveloped the wonderful dilapidated structure into the most unique and historic building it is today. Thank you so very much for his effort.
Signed, Charles Countee

Father's Voice
Preserving History in Shaw

There is a five-story brick building at 1816 Twelfth Street, in the Shaw neighborhood, that I have come to know well. Nearly a century ago, when the historic building first opened its doors in 1912, segregation was the word of the day. At the time, it was the first full-service YMCA facility dedicated to the black community.

By the time I became involved in 1987, the building was vacated and in serious disrepair after efforts by the YMCA failed to raise the necessary funds to keep the building open. In 2001 and today, after more than thirteen years of planning and work, the building has been restored and renovated and is called the Thurgood Marshall Center for Service and Heritage.

How did I become involved? And what was my role? As with most things in my life, my work with the Thurgood Marshall Center unfolded over the years. At the outset, I had no idea what I was getting into.

__The Twelfth Street YMCA__

The building's significance lies, first, in its rich history. For much of the twentieth century, the Twelfth Street building was home to a black YMCA chapter begun in 1853 by Anthony Bowen. It had a swimming pool, full gym and track, classrooms, bedrooms, and conference rooms. The center not only provided significant social and cultural activities for the surrounding communities; it was also the site of planning meetings during the Civil Rights Movement. A number of great African-American artists and leaders spent time there, including Duke Ellington and Thurgood Marshall.

In the late 1950s, schools and neighborhoods across the country began a messy and incomplete process of racial integration. While integration was clearly a hopeful step in our country's history, it had some unfortunate side effects. Whereas middle-class black families previously had no choice but to live in all-black neighborhoods and send their kids to all-black schools, integration afforded them more options. In moving to areas with better resources, middle-class African-Americans sometimes left behind increasingly impoverished neighborhoods.

During segregation, the Shaw neighborhood had become a thriving cultural center for the black community. Now, integration gave middle-class black families the freedom to move north from the Shaw area, to neighborhoods with better schools. The resulting economic depression in Shaw was likely one reason the Twelfth Street YMCA gradually ran low on funds and fell into disrepair. By 1982, it had to close its doors altogether.

__My Involvement__

In December 1987, my phone rang. It was Fred Taylor, a friend of mine and executive director of For Love of Children (FLOC).[65] I had worked closely with Fred during my years as an administrator at the FLOC Learning Center.

"I have an idea to discuss with you," he told me. The Twelfth Street YMCA was hoping to sell its building, he said. He described how some in the community were concerned that the historic building would be torn down for the sake of development. A newly formed organization was exploring options for buying the historic building, restoring it, and saving it from redevelopment that would not preserve its heritage. This organization—called the Shaw Heritage Trust—wanted to partner with another significant nonprofit in the effort.

Meanwhile, FLOC was outgrowing its current offices and wanted to move to a new space. Fred described how the Shaw Heritage Trust had contacted FLOC and a number of other nonprofit organizations about partnering with them. FLOC decided to apply and was selected by the Trust. Did this proposal hold any promise? Fred wondered if I might help FLOC in assessing the viability of the idea.

At the time of his phone call, I was just getting started in my work with the Rolling Ridge Retreat House. I wasn't sure how much energy I could dedicate to other projects, but I agreed to join Fred and a few others at a breakfast to explore the proposal further. That breakfast was the beginning of my involvement in a redevelopment effort that took longer than any of us imagined. During 1988, while most of my time was dedicated to Rolling Ridge, I worked about ten hours a week trying to evaluate what it would take to buy and renovate the historic building on Twelfth Street. I brought in architectural and construction firms for their assessment, attended meetings, wrote budgets, and researched a plan for purchasing the building.[66]

For the next thirteen years, I continued to work on the project, eventually increasing my time to thirty to forty hours a week. I won't go into all the details of what the project entailed, but I will say that, with one problem after another, there were many times we wondered if we'd have to drop the whole idea.

First, the Shaw Heritage Trust had to convince the YMCA not to sell the building to developers—who would likely pay a good price for it. To this end, the Trust sued the YMCA to prevent the sale. They uncovered a covenant written into the deed that stated the building was to be indefinitely dedicated to the benefit of "colored men." The two organizations settled outside of court, and the Shaw Heritage Trust was given a certain amount of time to detail a redevelopment plan.

FLOC and the Shaw Heritage Trust joined forces to form a new organization.[67] I did a significant amount of the research and work necessary to achieve 501(c)(3) tax-exempt status. This, too, proved difficult, as the government was slow to approve a nonprofit whose primary purpose was the ownership and preservation of a building.

The biggest challenge was raising the money necessary for the redevelopment plan. Originally, we estimated that the entire project would be completed by 1991, and cost three and half million dollars. In the end, we did not finish work on the building until the year 2000, and over the course of the project, spent six million dollars, partly due to the rise in construction costs in the 1990s.

The Shaw Heritage Trust suggested renaming the building, in part because it might help in our fundraising efforts—and chose the name of a prominent African-American with a historical connection to the Twelfth Street YMCA. When we finally opened the doors of the Thurgood Marshall Center for Service and Heritage in April 2000, I felt deep satisfaction.

♣

I was quite drawn to this project as unique, with benefits for the Shaw neighborhood, for the wider African-American community, and for FLOC. Preserving a building so deeply rooted in the history of the African-American struggle was a very worthwhile effort.

The building had a history of serving the community, and with our plan for redevelopment, it would continue to do so. The ground floor has become home to the FLOC Learning Center. On the main floor, photographs hang in a Heritage Center, telling the dynamic story of the YMCA building and the Shaw neighborhood. The main level also has a gym, dining room, kitchen, and conference rooms. Smaller nonprofits have offices on a third floor. And the top two stories have become the new location for FLOC's offices.

FLOC, which provides various services and programs for children and families, obviously benefits from the new and larger location for its offices, but I see other benefits for the organization as well. FLOC was started in 1965 by a compassionate group of people, mostly from white and middle-class backgrounds, but it has become more racially diverse in the years since. Increasingly, FLOC has hired staff and recruited board members from the African-American community. From my perspective, moving its offices to the Thurgood Marshall Center was one way to build an even greater connection to the African-American experience.

During my years with the Thurgood Marshall Center, my kids often complained of not knowing what to say when they were asked, "What does your dad do?" My role in the project *was* unique—and certainly hard for a child to explain.

I began as a consultant of sorts, helping FLOC evaluate and develop a vision and plan for the project. But my role grew. I became a hub, a point person with connections to all the groups involved: architects, construction managers, lawyers, FLOC, the Shaw Heritage Trust, and the collaborative non-profit they formed together.[68]

Even though my "hub" role was significant, I didn't consider myself a prominent leader. I worked mostly in the background while folks like Fred Taylor, Norris Dodson, and Charles Countee held the lime light.[69]

I very much enjoyed the work. I valued the close working relationships I developed with FLOC and Shaw Heritage Trust leaders and board members. Many of these were interracial relationships, giving me the opportunity to grow in my awareness of race relations. Because of all the groups involved, I certainly encountered conflict and sometimes helped facilitate communication between parties. I loved the challenge of enabling the different organizations to work together.

I was constantly learning new things. I especially enjoyed the window I got into the nature of different professions. I worked closely with architects and engineers in designing the building's renovations. I collaborated with lawyers in developing loan documents and organizational bylaws, negotiating zoning issues, financing the building, and seeking historic approvals. I also worked closely with the construction manager, a wonderful man named Jair Lynch.[70] While the project took much longer than I ever anticipated, it was stimulating and enriching work, and I enjoyed it.

__*Today*__

My disappointments with the project—and there were a few—had mostly to do with how things unfolded as the construction finished. In 2000 and the year following, FLOC and other smaller nonprofits moved into the building. The Thurgood Marshall Center Trust developed plans for operating and maintaining the building. It was exciting to see the building finally bustling with activity.

But in my final year with the project, I became aware of two conflicting cultures with two different visions for the building's purpose and maintenance. Those who had envisioned the project in its early years had assumed a low-budget, "homeowner" model of operation, in which the building's users would do much of the caretaking and maintenance. For example, FLOC employees would empty their own trash cans and sweep the floors. This was a culture of doing more with less and giving minimal priority to physical presentation.

Instead, the culture that emerged in the Thurgood Marshall Center gave priority to the image of both the organization and the building. To show due respect to the African-American heritage the building represented, the Thurgood Marshall Center Trust hired the people and services necessary for a polished image: a well-paid executive director and high-quality caretakers. They hired a building management team that provided security and cleaning services. I was afraid that the layers of overhead needed to preserve this level of presentation far exceeded the organization's capacity to pay.

In 2001, my work with the project was winding down. I phased out and turned most of my remaining responsibilities over to the newly hired executive director.[71] Today, in 2005, the building is still in great shape, but FLOC has run into significant financial problems. The forty-year-old nonprofit is downsizing and restructuring and may move out of the Thurgood Marshall Center altogether. This is clearly disappointing to me. I had hoped our vision for the project would prove sustainable.[72]

It appears that the organizational structure we had originally envisioned for the Thurgood Marshall Center is dissolving. Even so, I remain hopeful that other groups might replace FLOC and that the Thurgood Marshall Center will continue to serve the community in decades to come.

An important historical building has been saved. It still provides the community with a restored gym, a hallway, and a lobby area. The Heritage Center, a room on the main floor, is furnished to reflect the building's earlier era and will continue to develop a collection of old photographs and relics from the building, the neighborhood, and the larger African-American community. Even as the organizational structure changes, these will remain and continue to capture the sentiments and history of a dynamic African-American community in the nation's capital.

june 25, 2005

"If love is measured in bread," I said to Dad recently, "then you're doing pretty well." We have had an almost constant supply of homemade bread for months now, including a loaf that arrived in the mail from California. Amazing how many people still take the time for mixing and rising, kneading and baking.

Time has taken on new meaning for me during these weeks. In some senses, time matters so much less—I am the least busy I have ever been in my life. I have spent countless hours simply sitting in a room with Dad, keeping him company while he dozes in and out of conversation. In another sense, time is as precious as ever. We know our days together are few.

This week, Dad feels weaker still and comments that he's not processing things as quickly. This is likely both a sign of disease and a side effect of his medications. His liver continues to expand, and the edema (fluid retention) below his waist remains a problem. All this gives his body a very strange shape: thin arms, gaunt face, swollen abdomen, and chubby legs.

We open our doors to an almost daily stream of friends and family. Children sit with their parents on the couch and peer timidly at this kind and very ill man they have known, some of them all their lives. He sits in a padded recliner to ease his pain and smiles warmly at them.

"See my arms?" he says, rolling up his T-shirt sleeve. "They're so skinny, hardly more than skin and bones." I remember as a kid asking him again and again to make a muscle. My brothers and I would *ooh* and *ahh* at his biceps, well-cultivated by his boyhood on the farm and physical labor in the years since. Now they are a third the size of mine.

"But see how pudgy I am down here?" he asks the children, touching his legs. He pulls up the lower hem of his pants, revealing bloated ankles and calves. "There is a lot of fluid that gets stuck in the lower half of my body. Here," he says, "come touch them."

His favorite outfit these days—striped "putter pants" (as Mom calls them) and a royal blue tee shirt—disguise his disproportionate figure and bring out the blue in his eyes. Though the disease has altered his body and the loom of death has deepened his spirit, there is no mistake: Dad is still very much Dad. Last Sunday, Jason, Ryan, Hannah, and I were driving back from a gathering of Dad's brothers and families, bringing with us food and messages of love. On the way home in the car, Jason sent a "Happy Father's Day" text message to my parents' cell phone.

After several unsuccessful attempts at retrieving it, my dad asked Jason if he thought there would be cell phones in heaven. "Yes," said Jason. "And you better figure out how to use them before you get there!"

(Please understand, we laugh and cry in the same breath.)

So we have our bits of humor and our moments of deep joy. But, all in all, the days are edged with grief and frustration. Dad struggles with restlessness and anxiety, a "cabin fever" of sorts, and is trying both conventional and herbal remedies to calm his body and mind. If he's not restless, he's drowsy, and sometimes he's both at the same time.

After years of *do*-ing and planning, it is quite an adjustment to learn to *be* in the moment and have no future to plan for. Perhaps this is the hardest part for a man who has spent his life working on projects and playing with his kids but almost never sitting around. Even on family trips when Ryan, Jason, and I were young, I cannot remember Dad engaging in the activity I imagine most people do while on vacation: doing nothing. Instead, he was always planning the next step of the journey or organizing a basketball game.

Now, he is capable of very little. He rotates between bed and recliner, dining room table and wheel chair, and he never seems quite satisfied with his new choice of venue. Just this week, Dad was lying in bed, so I crawled up next to him. His eyes were closed. I did not think he was listening as Garrison Keillor spoke from the tape recorder, telling a story about children in Lake Wobegon. A few short weeks after school lets out for the summer, Keillor described, the kids flop down on the couch at home and sing out, "I'm BORED! This is BORING!"

At which point Dad, with his eyes still closed, said flatly in a raspy voice, "You could say the same thing about this room."

Before I knew what was happening, there we were. A weak and dying man and his daughter, lying flat on our backs, staring at the ceiling, and singing out: "I'm BORED! This is BORING!"

I laughed and laughed. Oh, Dad.

Even while grieving all that he is losing, Dad has started talking about his readiness to have this thing called death come and take him. This is especially hard for Mom, who would, of course, like him here as long as possible. I don't think ever in their married life have their journeys been so intertwined and so different at the same time. Dad is preparing to die, while Mom is wishing he wouldn't and preparing to survive without him.

So we adjust daily to each new stage. We rearrange furniture as needs change: Jason and I lowered my parents' bed to make it easier for Dad to get in and out. We made

room for a wheel chair and bedside table delivered today.
We play, we sit, we learn to be. We are held, kneaded,
cared for, changed. . . . We rise and we fall. Like bread.

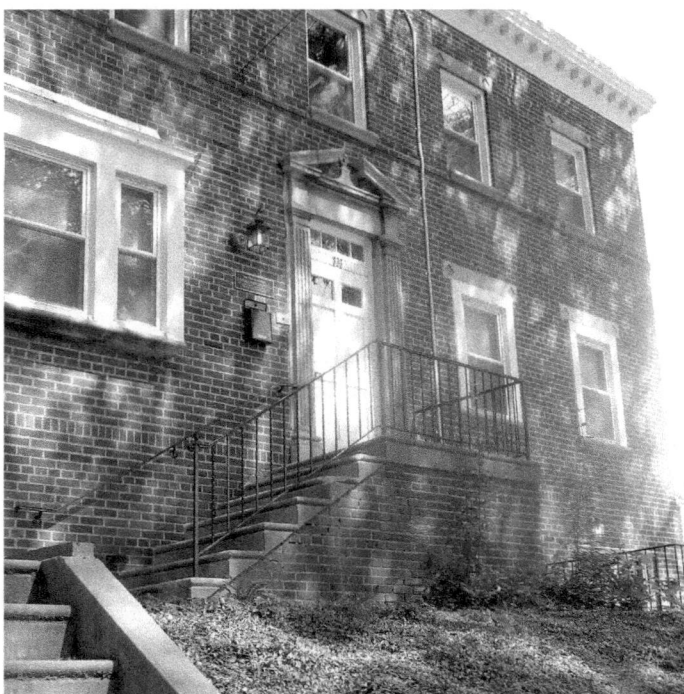

Several months before the Washington Community Scholars' Center (formerly WSSY) moved into the recently renovated house on Taylor Street, a plaque appeared by the front door, giving the new WCSC student house a name. Photo credit: Emily Benner

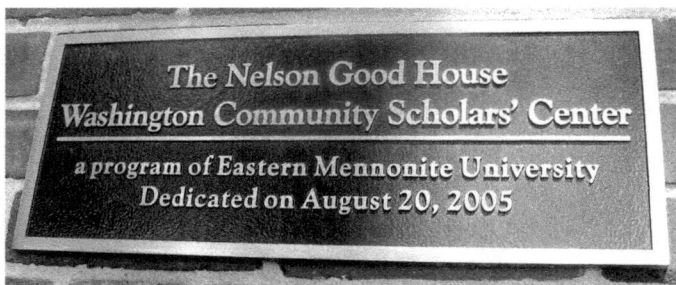

The Nelson Good House
Washington Community Scholars' Center

a program of Eastern Mennonite University
Dedicated on August 20, 2005

Chapter 7

Washington Community Scholars' Center

Daughter's Voice
Final Projects

Dad was not one to complain about physical pain. He rarely answered the question of "How are you?" with anything other than "Fine," "Really well," or "Great," when I got him on the phone, preferring to direct the conversation to me and my doings. Whenever I called home in January 2005, however, and asked Dad how he was doing, he responded with an unexpected, "Not very well, actually."

By the second week of January, Dad was on pain medication and spending hours of his day resting on a twin mattress in my parents' living room. The doctors believed he had a herniated disc in his back that would correct itself with time. From his spot on the living room floor, Dad continued to manage his various involvements, most notably his work coordinating the renovation of a new house for the WSSY/WCSC program.[73]

175

Dad's back started hurting in December 2004, right around the time of Ryan and Hannah's wedding. They were married New Year's Eve, in Goshen, Indiana. I was among the friends and family who gathered around them in a semi-circle, like two open palms, and afterward filled ourselves with salad, lasagna, cheesecake, and coffee.

At the service, Mom, Dad, and Hannah's parents each blessed the bride and groom with words of hope and welcome. Later, Ryan and Hannah gave me a photo of Dad at the mic, and whenever I look at it, I swear my heart gives a short, irregular squeeze. There's no need to hear his words to understand that this was one of Dad's toe-to-head joyful moments; you can see it in his eyes. He is sixty years old and looks healthy enough to hike a mountain.

The next afternoon, Jason, Bryn, Dad, and I went bowling. The man with the injured back—we assumed he'd strained it setting up chairs and tables for the wedding—won, hands down. He never told us he had taken bowling classes in college.

Some people think of us as an athletic family. Dad, us kids, and various combinations of our friends and neighbors could often be found playing basketball in the alley and—if we found enough grass or a spot on the beach—soccer, volleyball, ultimate frisbee, or football, while Mom (God bless her) was all too often inside, chopping vegetables and stirring soup for our evening meal. Still, I don't remember bowling as a family before this particular New Year's, but it was the last sport we enjoyed together with Dad.

Later that night, Ryan and Hannah joined the rest of us for supper at the guest house where we were staying. We finished our food and lingered around the table, talking, laughing, shifting our hips under full stomachs. The phone rang. It was Dad's brother, Luke. The man with the injured back left the room to take the call. When he returned, he sat quietly in his seat at the end of the table. The rest of us were very involved in our con-

versation until Hannah—I remember clearly it was Hannah—
turned to him and saw something quivering behind his eyes.

"Nelson, is everything okay?"

Dad was not generally a crier, but he responded to Hannah's question with heavy sobs. His shoulders shook with the
weight of them, his head leaning down toward his hands on the
table, as though hanging from an invisible thread. We knew
that his mother had been admitted at the hospital just before
the wedding. They had now, he said, diagnosed her with cancer. Pancreatic cancer. The doctors didn't think she had long to
live.

Her twenty-one grandchildren called her Grandma Good.
She was Ruth, the woman in a cape dress and covering who
made the best donuts I've ever eaten and never stopped quilting, even when she had seven boys at home, a large garden, and
piles of mending, cooking, and cleaning to tend to. Even when
the chicken house burned, then the tractor. Even when her
boys left home and spanned the globe with their service work
and travel. Even when Grandpa was struck with Alzheimer's
and taken from her one week at a time. Grandma was always
quilting. And now she was dying, and my dad sat at the end of
the table, sobbing.

Looking back, this moment marked the beginning of the
year to come. It was New Year's Day, but that is not what I
mean. What I mean is the air around us, the way it shifted pal-
pably with the news; the way our wedding moods settled into
the pits of our stomachs, making room for the confusion,
anger, and sorrow of death's coming shadow. What I mean is
Dad's vulnerable, shaking shoulders, and the pain aching
silently in his lower back.

Mom, Dad, and I decided to drive through the night,
reaching the hospital in Lancaster the next morning for a meeting with his brothers and their wives. Dad did not sleep well in
the car. He stretched and re-folded his hurting body, adjusting
his pillow against the window.

Grandma died in March. We buried her at Hammer Creek Mennonite, next to Grandpa who had died three years earlier. Dad watched the funeral the next day, videotaped, from his bed in D.C.

♣

Nearly twenty-five years after helping to found the program and then serving as one of its directors (or "coordinators," as he preferred to call himself), Dad was invited to join the WSSY board in 1999. Over the next few years, he was instrumental in evaluating whether to move the program from the original house on South Dakota Avenue to a new location and then overseeing the renovation of an abandoned apartment building he'd located for the purpose.

Current WCSC director Kimberly Schmidt remembers Dad's initial offer to help. *I will never forget calling Nelson to confer about relocation difficulties,* she wrote in the WCSC newsletter. *In his slow, deliberate way he responded, "That's a nut I'd like to help you crack." From that day forward, Nelson led the way in presenting financial plans to EMU, tracking down possible properties in a number of neighborhoods, researching owners of delinquent properties, and gathering support from local alumni.*[74]

Dad's leadership in solving WCSC's relocation quandary required some of his most practiced skills: networking between talented folks, envisioning the use of physical space, thinking financially, and getting down-and-dirty in construction work.

In some senses, it was a grace that Dad could be involved in this project before he died. I say this mostly because Dad might have said something similar. *Grace* was one of his favorite words. The project was a grace, he might have said, because it re-involved him in a program he helped to birth and circled him back to other pieces of his life, as though taking him on a road trip through his years in the city, revisiting all the people he had met along the way. To make the renovation possible, he tapped shoulders and made phone calls. He pooled together his own skills with those of people he knew—through his work with Friendship Flat, Rolling Ridge, House Church, and the Thurgood Marshall Center.

Jay Good, who had worked closely with Dad in the early days of Rolling Ridge, now slept many nights at my parents' house while managing the renovations of the new WCSC house, returning to his home in Annville, Pennsylvania, on weekends. After a long day of work, he would sit in a chair in the living room, while Dad lay on his mattress on the floor, and discuss the day's progress.

Dad had a hard time letting go of this job. A few weeks after his back pain led to a shocking cancer diagnosis, Mom sat with him in a doctor's waiting room—a common pastime for us in those days. He was trying to decide whether to stay involved in the WCSC project as much as he was able or whether to extract himself altogether. He carried a strong sense of responsibility, mixed up with his love and pride for the program, and he needed help releasing it. Mom listened thoughtfully. Ultimately, he decided on the latter, left the work in the hands of the team he had assembled, and turned his attention to his disease, his family, and the possibility of his imminent death.

Even so, Dad remained interested in the happenings at 836 Taylor Street. Once, on the way home from a radiation appointment, we stopped by the work site to check on the progress. Dad hobbled around wooden planks, cinder blocks, and mounds of dirt in his slippers, a urine bag looped over his left crutch. It strikes me now how totally un-self-conscious he was, mostly oblivious to the fact that his pee was hanging out in a bag by his side. Maybe if we all cared less about our facades, our imperfections—our urine bags—we'd have more energy left over for changing the world.

♣

Sometime during spring 2005, EMU president Loren Swartzendruber came to my parents' home in D.C. to visit with my dad. Loren's job on this particular day was a challenging one. He had come to ask for Dad's approval of the proposed name for the new WCSC building: the Nelson Good House.

Anyone who has worked with my dad knows that he was wary of anything that brought the spotlight to himself. He worried that someone else might be more deserving of the honor, or that people who came across the "Nelson Good House" might wrongly attribute too much credit to him. Perhaps it was just Mennonite modesty. But I believe Dad also understood, profoundly, that raising up communities and programs with his life would impact the world in far more significant ways than raising up his own name ever could.

Loren's conversation with Dad was fruitful. He listened to Dad's concerns, affirming his contribution to the university and to the hundreds of students who have passed through the WSSY/WCSC program since its inception. Loren expressed his deep wish that Dad would be well again and could be part of the building's dedication in August the same year. With some mixture of reluctance and satisfaction, Dad consented to the naming of the building, and whenever he mentioned it in the months that followed, he chuckled in embarrassment.

When Dad died in July, the Nelson Good House was still five months from completion. A month later, the building dedication happened in his honor but without him there. He would have loved to see it today, bustling with the noise and clutter of college students.

Father's Voice
WSSY . . . Again

For the first decade following my retirement from WSSY in 1987, I had very little connection with the program. I don't remember being invited back to give presentations in seminar or to serve on the board. In reality, I felt somewhat cut off, which was confusing and hard for me after being so deeply involved.

In 1999, I was recruited to join the WSSY advisory board. It felt very good to be back in close touch with the program, helping to review issues and solve problems. Eastern Mennonite University was still strongly committed to WSSY, as evident in their willingness to hire staff with strong credentials. The board began a process of looking ahead to WSSY's future. What changes would strengthen the program in the years to come?

In evaluating the future direction of an organization, I find it helpful to review several pieces separately. One is the structure and design of the program and a second is whether an organization's staff are well-matched for its demands. A third important piece—sometimes given too little weight—involves evaluating a program's location and facility. Well-planned physical space and location can do a lot to shape and strengthen a program.

__The Facility Question__

WSSY has continued using the house on South Dakota Avenue all these years, primarily because it was inexpensive.[75] But, in a number of ways, the house has not been an ideal location for the WSSY/WCSC program. It is located along a busy street, which makes it isolated and difficult to feel a part of the neighborhood. Public transportation is accessible but inconvenient. What's more, the house is not compliant with city regulations: It is not zoned correctly and does not meet building codes for student housing.

In June 2003, I was assigned the task of reviewing the facility question—assessing whether WCSC should upgrade the existing house or consider moving to a new location. The answer was not clear. Making improvements and zoning changes at the current location would cost considerable money. It seemed unwise to invest so much in a house that already had so many shortcomings. Moving to a new location, in a city where housing prices are very high and rising, would undoubtedly cost even more. It became my assessment and hope that, in the long run, a new location would be of great benefit to EMU.

Finding a new place that met our requirements would not be easy. We wanted a house that could fit ten to fifteen students, in a location that was residential, zoned correctly, and near a subway station. I identified four target neighborhoods and began scouting. It was winter—late 2003. I worked block by block, sometimes on foot and sometimes in my car, looking for large abandoned houses or small apartment buildings with their windows boarded up.

When I did find an abandoned building that had potential, I would search tax records for the owner's name and address. Usually these buildings were not on the market. They were simply sitting there along the street, boarded up and empty. My goal was to find an owner who was willing to sell.

Months passed, and I hadn't had any luck. Then, one day, I was driving around a neighborhood that I'd already searched once. In my earlier search, I had decided that the apartment buildings there were a little too small, without space enough on their lots to build an addition. But this time, as I drove along Taylor Street, I happened to notice one boarded-up building that I had overlooked before: 836 Taylor Street. It had a basement apartment, which allowed for more space, and the lot was big enough for an addition off the back. Could this be the one?

I searched the Internet to find an address for the owner and asked our realtor, to send him a letter. After a few weeks with no response, I decided to go in person to the owner's house. His young-adult daughter answered the door.

"Is Mr. Kenneth McDow home?" I asked her.

"I'm sorry. He's not here."

I explained briefly who I was and left my phone number. To my pleasant surprise, Mr. McDow called me. But he was not interested in selling; he had plans to renovate the building for his daughter when she graduated from college.

"The party I represent will pay generously," I promised.

Mr. McDow agreed to at least walk me through the building. Within the week, EMU submitted an offer of $330,000.

"Well, to change our plans and buy a condominium for our daughter," he said, "will cost us more than that." EMU increased its offer to $350,000, which was very generous for that neighborhood and the condition of the building. Even at the higher price, I believed this was a good buy for EMU, because a building that fit the program's unique needs was a rare find. And—to my great delight—Mr. McDow accepted the offer. It was April 14, 2004, when we settled, and I felt great.

__Renovations and the Future__

As I have often done throughout my life, I drew on my various contacts to pull off the building's purchase and renovation. Norris Dodson, from the Thurgood Marshall Center, was our realtor. David Conrad, who had worked with me on the Rolling Ridge Retreat House, agreed to do the architectural planning. An old friend and member of House Church named John Swarr, who works as a general construction manager, would be a consultant. And Jay Good, from the early days at Rolling Ridge, became the onsite construction manager.

Today,[76] the building is still amid renovations, but it already looks far different from the abandoned building I first walked through in March 2004. The renovated building will house up to fifteen students, with large dining and living room areas, a classroom to accommodate up to twenty-five people, a study and computer room, and an office for staff.

Many WSSY alumni remember eating breakfast at the old South Dakota Avenue house and hanging out around the "island" in the kitchen; they will be happy to know that the new kitchen has a similar island. This house, unlike the old one, will be handicapped-accessible. Completion is scheduled for October 2005.[77]

The WSSY/WCSC program is notable for its longevity. It has been around for nearly thirty years and appears to have

many good years still in store. It has been reshaped and revital-
ized over time so that it continues to be relevant to students
today—and it has likely survived so long, in part, because of its
openness to change. Even though pieces of the program are different from when I served as one of its coordinators during the
'70s and '80s, the basic thrust is the same.

It appears that I will not be around to see the students move
in and make the new WCSC house their home, which, of
course, saddens me deeply. But it is something of a gift that the
opportunity arose for me—at what we now know is the end of
my life—to be once again so closely involved with the
WSSY/WCSC program. I have confidence in the gifts and
commitment of the many good people who will carry the vision of the program into the coming years.

EPILOGUE:
A DAUGHTER'S
REFLECTIONS

On the last day of June 2005, Fred Taylor came to visit my dad. I was doing something in the next room when Dad called me in.

"This wise man is saying something," he said to me with a smile.

Fred had said Dad's life truly exemplified "servant leadership," and Dad wanted him to explain what he meant.

"A servant leader," said Fred, "is someone with a vision." He lifted his hands out in front of his face as though shaping the air into an amorphous vision-cloud. "He looks at a situation, sees a possibility, and sees all that needs to be done to make it happen." Fred explained that a servant leader doesn't just hold up visions for others to follow. He's on the ground, taking care of details, doing concrete work—sometimes with a hammer, sometimes with a computer spreadsheet—subtly moving people toward the vision.

It was amazing, really, to see these two white-haired men talk—one with a full, healthful face and deep southern accent, the other leaning back in his creaky recliner to reduce the swelling in his legs, small bowls hollowed into his cheeks, his subtle Pennsylvania Dutch undertones betraying his rural past. They discussed their work together in the city and their cooperative ideas for change.

I believe Fred is right: Dad was a practical visionary, a servant leader. He had a vision for creating shared retreat space at Rolling Ridge and, to make it happen, he once literally found himself up to his waist in mud. He imagined an experiential education program for college students and, to make it happen, found himself changing light bulbs and negotiating the tedious details of various internship arrangements. Dad was a "big picture" guy who also handled the nuts and bolts.

Dad also had a profound ability to criticize a project while at the same time pouring his time and energy into it. I have seen folks discuss all day long the imperfections of an idea and never follow through with it. Dad understood no model was perfect, but that did not keep him from moving forward with some notion of a better option—whether it was Friendship Flat, the Learning Center, or Rolling Ridge. He held his critiques in one hand and a hammer in the other.

♣

I usually try to meet problems with solutions. Last year, books that my housemates and I had stored in our basement began to mold. I hunted the Internet for a used dehumidifier, and then drove across town to buy one up from another young woman. Back at home, I carried it down to the basement and plugged it in. It whirred happily, sucking moisture from the air and dripping it into a plastic bucket which we used for laundry, dumped on the garden, or simply emptied into an outdoor drain and down into the pipes below.

Even with big things, so huge and terrible, there is nothing my small hands could do to solve them, I sometimes find myself trying. For weeks after September 11, 2001, I met other Eastern Mennonite University students outside the school library and carpooled to the town square, where we joined other bewildered Americans on a street corner, holding signs that read "No War, No Retaliation" and "We Mourn ALL Killing."

Grief, I am discovering, is something entirely different. I can't solve grief with dehumidifiers. Nor address it with peace marches. Grief asks not that we *do*, but instead that we sit and explore all those spaces inside our minds and bodies where memories are stored. In the privacy of our homes and in the public space of funerals, it asks that we spend time in each of its rooms and hallways, feel its depths, scream, cry, sit in silence, and, occasionally, dance.

One week before Dad breathed his last, my mom and I were caring for him around the clock. On Wednesday, Ryan arrived by train from Indiana. Having him at home freed me to spend a much-needed night out with a friend. We went to see a film called *Rize*, which documents a grassroots dance movement in South Central Los Angeles. Young men and women, mostly living amid poverty, violence, and great difficulty, gather together and *krump*—they move their bodies with almost unbelievable speed and power, dancing out their youth and their anger with a ferocious dignity.

Alone in my room that night, I found myself doing a little of the same. I put in music and let tears and anger move my body, releasing grief like sweat from my pores.

One week later, early on the morning of July 13, 2005, Jason knocked on my bedroom door, waking me. "Dad just passed," he said. We gathered downstairs around his bed, Mom, Ryan, Jason, and I. His body was still warm. We told stories of the past week and before. We laughed and shed some tears. We touched him. I reached my hands in under his back where the flesh was still warm.

♣

People have said grief comes in waves. Some six months after the funeral, one rolled in without warning; I got pummeled.

At the time, I was working several part-time, temporary, and odd jobs. Some people had told me that they survived the terrible waves of sadness by keeping busy.

I suddenly felt unable to carry it all. I decided that one of my part-time jobs was wearing me out, that my time was too full and my energy too depleted. I needed to pay attention to my sadness, to slow down and "sit with the s---," as my friend Melody would say. I resigned.

I had the radio on as I stood in the shower one morning after turning in my resignation letter, uncomfortable with my choice to work less and feeling like a failure. A woman named Mary Cook was reading a three-minute essay, part of a National Public Radio series called "This I Believe." I stepped from the shower and stood, dripping in my towel, as I realized what Cook's essay was about. Her fiancé had died suddenly several years ago. In the months afterwards, she'd felt mortified and guilty for being so immobilized by her loss. She had worried that others would think her lazy.

"One very wise man once told me," I heard her say, "'You are not doing nothing. Being fully open to your grief may be the hardest work you ever do.'"[78]

I ran from the bathroom to write down her words.

During the first year after Dad's death, I learned to know someone new: my grieving self. I discovered my grieving self needed a lot of time alone. I sometimes tried to describe what I was going through to friends, but words felt superficial and— surprisingly—writing felt like a chore.

Perhaps silence comes first. Words must germinate like seeds, unseen beneath the dark soil of our inner gardens, later growing splendidly into tomatoes, green beans, and peppers. Maybe, I realized, my peppers would take time. Maybe the pages of this book are my peppers.

Over time, my grief became less like a bulldozer and more like a needy and unpredictable mutt who followed me every-where I went. Her presence became strangely comforting and so familiar that I sometimes forgot she was there—until I accidentally stepped backwards onto her tail, and she nipped me in the ankle, my eyes smarting unexpectedly from the pain.

The five and a half months between Dad's diagnosis and death changed me forever. I don't want to call it a *journey*—but a blundering. Our family's blundering through that liminal space was pain, and it was gift. I am endlessly grateful for the hours I spent with Dad in those final months. They were a long farewell, a chance to listen in depth to a man who has known me since birth, whose genes live on in my DNA, and whose story is inextricably intertwined with mine.

Being with my own dying father as he reflected on his adult life—and then listening to his voice again as I transcribed the audio-recordings of our conversations—was an intensely intimate experience. I thank you, dear reader, for letting me share pieces of it with you.

ACKNOWLEDGMENTS: A WORD OF THANKS

I must begin this page of gratitude by thanking my mom, Betty Wenger Good, without whose memory, emotional investment, ongoing encouragement, tireless work, and endless patience this project would have been impossible. Mom read drafts of every chapter more than twice. She sometimes stuck with me on the phone until well past her bedtime as we processed questions of wording and meaning, striving always for authenticity and accuracy, and sometimes disagreeing strongly regarding what that looked like.

Thanks also to my brothers and their partners—Ryan Good, Hannah Dueck, Jason Good, and Bryn Mullet Good—who also read chapter drafts, lost the same father I did, and taught me countless lessons about gratitude, grief, and good humor along the way.

Thanks to Dan Charles and Sara Wenger Shenk, whose careful reading of an early draft of the manuscript provided me with invaluable feedback and suggestions for improvement. Thanks to Cascadia publisher Michael A. King for encouraging me to submit the manuscript to his editorial council, nudging me to add more of my voice to it, and making publication as a book a real possibility. Head-to-toe thanks to Melody King and

Julie Kauffman, who lived with me while I tried to find a rhythm of writing, work, rest, and play that would sustain me, even through the hardest months of grief. And to the many friends who have asked for updates on this book's progress only to hear me say time and again (for nearly two years!) that I was almost finished, and whose words have propped up my lagging belief in myself as a writer.

Thanks to Tom Donlon for his book, *Faith Road to Rolling Ridge*, which proved an important resource in my writing and editing of the Rolling Ridge chapter. Thanks to Verle Headings for reading Dad's half of that chapter and suggesting corrections, to Fred Taylor who did the same for the chapters on the Learning Center and Thurgood Marshall Center, to countless others for answering my fact-checking e-mails and for responding to my call for photographs.

I am grateful, too, for the Philadelphia coffee shops where I spent many hours with my laptop, and especially for Kaffa Crossing, the Ethiopian café on Chestnut Street that became my "office space" of choice. The Virginia fruit farm of my aunt and uncle, Margaret and Samuel Johnson, also proved a fruitful place (no pun intended!) for a small chunk of the transcribing and writing, while I picked grapes for them in September 2005.

I finished the manuscript while living with Keith and Rachelle Lyndaker Schlabach at Rolling Ridge. My deepest appreciation for their hospitality at a time of significant transition in their own lives, and thanks, indeed, to everyone in the Rolling Ridge community who took me in for the summer, and fueled my writing with their memories and stories. I can't think of a better place to reflect on and write about my dad. (If my drafts weren't done on computer but written with pen and paper, my pages would smell of mountain dirt and wildflowers, of summer's relentless heat.)

And the grand finale: Thanks above all thanks go to the spectacular human being whose words compose half of this book and inspired the rest. Thank you, Dad, for your intentional and unmatched parenting, your constant affirmation, your servant leadership and humility, your gentle questions about the world and our roles in it; for your left-handed hook shot, your made-from-scratch macaroni and cheese, and, above all else, your deep-rooted ideals of selflessness and love. You were one hell of a dad. I love you.

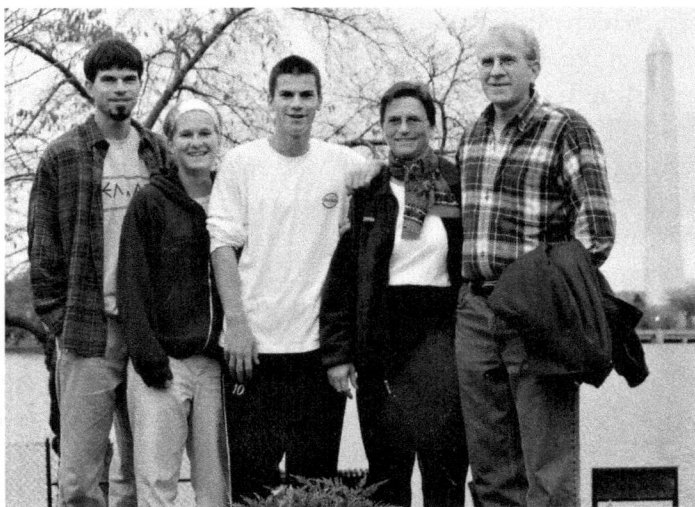

*Ryan, Deborah, Jason, Betty, and Nelson Good;
Thanksgiving 2001.*

Appendix A

TIME LINE FOR THE LIFE OF NELSON W. GOOD
MAY 16, 1944–JULY 13, 2005

May 16, 1944: born to Ira and Ruth Weaver Good in family farm house, Lititz, PA

June 1960: completed tenth grade (his last year of school) to work on the farm with his father

August 1964: enrolled at Eastern Mennonite College after completing GED

May 1968: earned BS in Sociology from Eastern Mennonite College

August 18, 1968: married Betty Wenger

September 1968–September 1970: moved to Washington, D.C., and volunteered with Eastern Mennonite Board of Missions and Charities (EMBMC) at *Friendship Flat*, which was a voluntary service unit and community center between 1966 and 1973

1970–1976: served as half-time administrator for EMBMC voluntary service units in Philadelphia, PA, and Washington, D.C.

Fall 1971: helped in founding and opening of the *FLOC Learning Center*

March 1973: became administrator of the *FLOC Learning Center*, a role he kept for 13 years

May 1973: earned Masters in Sociology, The Catholic University of America

February 1974: bought first home at 2720 Ontario Road, NW, Washington, D.C.

Spring 1975: participated in the first exploratory visit to a piece of land in West Virginia where the Rolling Ridge Study Retreat Community (RRSRC) would eventually form

August 1976–August 1977: was founder and coordinator for the first year of *Washington Study-Service Year* (WSSY, now WCSC), remaining in the role until 1987

Summer 1976: participated in camping trip to *Rolling Ridge*, Harpers Ferry, WV

1977: lease signed with Rolling Ridge Foundation for 130 acres of land for the *RRSRC*

January 13, 1978: birth of first child, Ryan Mathias

1978: joined *Community House Church* where he was a member until he died

October 6, 1980: birth of second child, Deborah Anna

May 1, 1982–October 1, 1982: family lived at *Rolling Ridge* while Nelson was on sabbatical from *FLOC Learning Center* and *WSSY*

April 29, 1983: birth of third child, Jason Lloyd

December 1985: bought and moved to 1800 Kenyon Street, NW, the home where Nelson was living when he died

December 1986: retired from *FLOC Learning Center*

Summer 1987: retired from *Washington Study-Service Year*

December 1987: became involved in project which is now the *Thurgood Marshall Center for Service and Heritage*

1988: construction of the retreat house at *RRSRC*

April 2000: dedication of the *Thurgood Marshall Center for Service and Heritage*

June 20, 2001: retired from his role at the *Thurgood Marshall Center*

1999–2005: served on advisory board of *Washington Study-Service Year* during which time the name was changed to Washington Community Scholars Center

June 2003: was assigned the task of reviewing the facility question for *WSSY/WCSC* by the board

April 4, 2004: new building bought by Eastern Mennonite University for *WCSC* at 836 Taylor Street, NE, Washington, D.C.

January 26, 2005: diagnosed with stage IV adrenocortical cancer

July 13, 2005: died at home in the early morning hours

August 20, 2005: dedication of the Nelson Good House for the *WCSC* program

January 2006: *WCSC* students moved into the Nelson Good House for the first time

This chronology was compiled with considerable help from Betty Wenger Good.

Appendix B

THE ORGANIZATIONS
IN THIS BOOK

Church of the Saviour

In the 1940s, Gordon and Mary Cosby founded an ecumenical Christian church called Church of the Saviour. The church understood Christian faith to involve both *inward* spiritual development and *outward* work in the world, and was very active in social causes. In addition to gathering for worship on Sunday mornings at 2025 Massachusetts Avenue in northwest Washington, D.C., members met in smaller *mission groups* during the week, which, over the years, were responsible for developing a number of nonprofit organizations in the city (see *For Love of Children,* below).

In 1977, Church of the Saviour divided into smaller sister churches—the "scattered community"—because of its growing size. While each of these congregations operates independently and has its own character, all of the sister churches share common history, values, and practices. For more information on the Church of the Saviour churches and ministries as they exist today, visit <www.inwardoutward.org>.

Church of the Saviour
2025 Massachusetts Ave NW
Washington, D.C. 20036
(202) 387-1617

Community House Church

Community House Church (CHC) began in the 1970s as a small, ecumenical house fellowship in the Mount Pleasant neighborhood of northwest Washington, D.C. The group eventually outgrew homes, and since the 1990s has rented space in a variety of locations for worship and Sunday school. Current members come from all over the D.C. metropolitan area.

Even as the church has changed over the years, several features have remained constant: a model of lay leadership, a monthly members meeting as the locus of pastoral care and decision-making, participation in bimonthly small groups, a practice of annual recommitment, and a high level of personal sharing. Currently the group has many connections to the Anabaptist tradition, including links with Mennonite Mutual Aid, Mennonite Central Committee, Mennonite universities, and local Mennonite churches, but as a congregation, remains nondenominational.

Because of CHC's informal organization and the group's shared and shifting leadership, CHC has neither a website nor official contact information. Those interested should contact this book's author through Cascadia Publishing House.

Eastern Mennonite Missions (formerly Eastern Mennonite Board of Missions and Charities or"Eastern Board")

Eastern Mennonite Missions is an Anabaptist missionary organization located in Lancaster County, Pennsylvania, and supported primarily by the churches of Lancaster Mennonite Conference. In its earlier incarnation as Eastern Board, the agency placed volunteers in a number of United States locations, including two volunteer houses in Washington, D.C. Between 1968 and 1970, Nelson and Betty Good served for two years as volunteers in one of the houses, called Friendship Flat. Today, Eastern Mennonite Missions' focus is mostly international, with missionary and service efforts in more than thirty countries. For more information on Eastern Mennonite Missions of today, visit <www.emm.org>.

Eastern Mennonite Missions
www.emm.org
53 West Brandt Blvd
PO Box 458
Salunga, PA 17538-0458
(717) 898-2251

Eastern Mennonite University (formerly Eastern Mennonite College)

Eastern Mennonite University (EMU) offers undergraduate, graduate, and seminary programs to more than 1,400 students annually. The school was founded in 1917 as a Bible academy on the hillside in Harrisonburg, Virginia, where it is still located today as a liberal arts university. EMU has roots in a Mennonite heritage and, as described in the school's identity statement, "emphasizes peacebuilding, creation care, experiential learning, and cross-cultural engagement." It continues to offer college credit to students completing the WCSC program begun by Nelson Good in 1976 (see below).

Eastern Mennonite University
www.emu.edu
1200 Park Road
Harrisonburg, VA 22802
(540) 432-4000

For Love of Children and the Learning Center

In 1965, a mission group from Church of the Saviour founded an organization focused on serving troubled families and at-risk children in Washington, D.C., and named it For Love of Children (FLOC). The nonprofit organization has advocated for changes in city policies relevant to the lives of children and families, while also providing a variety of housing, foster care, and educational services.

Over the years, a number of programs developed under the FLOC umbrella, including the FLOC Learning Center. Begun in 1971, the Learning Center was in operation for thirty-four years as an alternative day school for children with special needs. In 2005, financial challenges forced FLOC to close a number of its programs including the Learning Center, whose students were integrated into the public school system' special education programs. For more information on FLOC as it exists today, visit www.flocdc.org.

For Love of Children
www.flocdc.org
1763 Columbia Road, NW, First Floor
Washington, D.C. 20009
(202) 462-8686

Rolling Ridge Study Retreat Community

Rolling Ridge Study Retreat Community is a small intentional community and ecumenical retreat center located in the Blue Ridge Mountains on 1,400 wooded acres near Harpers Ferry, West Virginia. A community of volunteer "staff" live year-round in four houses arranged around a central garden; a fifth house was still under construction as of this publication.

On the opposite hillside from the community's homes are a meditation shelter, art cottage, and six-bedroom retreat house, which are frequented by small churches and other groups from Washington, D.C., and nearby. The residential community also organizes a number of retreat events throughout the year focusing on themes of spirituality, biblical studies, meditative arts, earthkeeping, peacemaking, and community.

Rolling Ridge Study Retreat Community
www.rollingridge.net
129 Jubilee Lane

Harpers Ferry, WV 25425
(304) 724-6653

Thurgood Marshall Center for Service and Heritage

The Thurgood Marshall Center for Service and Heritage is located in Washington, D.C.'s historic Shaw neighborhood. The building was formerly home to the Twelfth Street YMCA, the country's first full-service YMCA for African-Americans, which was an important fixture in the neighborhood. The building has received many influential visitors including Thurgood Marshall and Langston Hughes.

Several years after the YMCA closed in 1982 and the building fell into disrepair, several nonprofit organizations joined efforts to restore the historic structure and open its doors anew. The process took more than a decade, but when renovations were complete, the newly opened Thurgood Marshall Center became home to several organizations, including For Love of Children and the Learning Center (see above), and a venue for community gatherings and events. In the years since, the Learning Center has closed and FLOC has moved out of the building, while other nonprofits have moved in. The Thurgood Marshall Center for Service and Heritage continues to stand as a testimony to the rich heritage of D.C.'s African-American community.

Thurgood Marshall Center Trust Inc.
www.thurgoodmarshallcenter.org
1816 12th St., N.W.
Washington, D.C. 20009
(202) 462-8314

Washington Community Scholars' Center (formerly WSSY)

Washington Community Scholars' Center (WCSC) is an experiential learning program of Eastern Mennonite University. Students accepted into the program spend one or two semesters living in a group house in Washington, D.C., taking classes at a local university, and interning at organizations in the city. WCSC was begun in 1976 as a year-long program called Washington Study-Service Year. More than thirty years after its founding, WCSC continues to impact the lives of students through community-living, hands-on internship experiences, exposure to a variety of urban issues, and a weekly seminar class that proposes to integrate the students' experiences with their classroom learning.

Washington Community Scholars Center
www.emu.edu/wcsc
836 Taylor Street, NE
Washington, D.C. 20017

Notes

1. These communities included Friendship Flat, the FLOC Learning Center, Community House Church, Washington Study-Service Year, and Rolling Ridge, all described later in this book.

2. The project was supervised and funded by the Eastern Mennonite Board of Missions and Charities, commonly called simply "Eastern Board."

3. Eastern Mennonite Board of Missions and Charities or Eastern Board, placed conscientious objectors in volunteer placements—domestically and abroad—during the Vietnam War. In Washington, D.C., they founded a community center called Friendship Flat at 1425 W Street, staffed by volunteers like my mom and dad.

4. The decision to close the unit at 1425 W Street was made by its founding organization, Eastern Board, for multiple reasons: Dad's analysis of the project's flaws, staff turnover, and difficulty finding good volunteer leadership, among others. After Friendship Flat closed, Dad continued to work for Eastern Board for three more years as half-time administrator for their remaining voluntary service unit in the city, located on South Dakota Avenue in northeast Washington.

5. Janet Liechty, July 2005.

6. page 8

7. page 9, italics mine

8. *The Institution as Servant,* page 1

9. Janet Liechty, Eulogy, July 2005.

10. In Chapter 4, Dad tells of his involvement in founding and developing Rolling Ridge Study Retreat Community, located near Harpers Ferry, West Virginia.

11. *The Servant as* Leader, page 10

12. See Chapter 7

13. From 1970 to 1976, Dad worked half-time as the in-town supervisor for Friendship Flat and a second voluntary service unit, located on South Dakota Avenue. Both units were projects of the Eastern Mennonite Board of Missions and Charities (Eastern Board).

14. As described in Chapter 1, Eastern Board closed Friendship Flat in 1973. Two years later, it closed its second unit, on South Dakota Avenue. This would eventually put Dad out of a job, as he was the in-town supervisor for these two units, but it also gave him a potential location for his envisioned student program. Eastern Board agreed to keep the house on South Dakota Avenue rather than putting it up for sale, while Dad and Gerry Meck worked to gain EMC's approval. For the first several years, EMC rented the house from Eastern Board at minimal cost. Eventually, EMC would buy the building in 1979 for a very modest price of $50,000.

15. In 1973, Dad had begun working part-time as the administrator of a school called the Learning Center. He tells this story in Chapter 3.

16. This was the only year that a faculty member lived in the house with the WSSY students.

17. The new building, since named the Nelson Good House in his honor, was dedicated in August 2005. Students moved in at the beginning of 2006. In Chapter 7, Dad tells his story of searching the neighborhoods of D.C. for a building suitable for the program, and finding this one—an abandoned apartment building—on Taylor Street.

18. "Are any among you sick? They should call for the elders of the church and have them pray over them, anointing them with oil in the name of the Lord."

19. Luke 6:20-35.

20. The Church of the Saviour still exists today, not as one centralized church but as a "diaspora" of smaller congregations. Gordon Cosby, the church's founder, emphasized that smaller is better—that churches with fewer members are often more alive and active, and so in 1976, after thirty years of meeting as one congregation, the church divided itself into six different groups which still meet today.

21. FLOC was initially begun by members of the Church of the Saviour who returned from participating in Freedom Marches in the South asking, "What can we do to free the children of Washington?" Fred Taylor became FLOC's director early on and encouraged participation beyond the Church of the Saviour's members. By the time the Learning Center opened in 1971, folks from a number of D.C. churches were involved in the organization.

22. The language of "call" was common among those familiar with the Church of the Saviour. They understood their spiritual journeys to be both inward *and* outward and believed that God calls humans personally and collectively to act in the world.

23. After significant effort, my friend's group has successfully opened a clinic in the neighborhood, called Puentes de Salud.

24. FLOC's primary objective was to create healthy alternatives to Junior Village and, if at all possible, to keep families intact. They created foster homes for sibling sets and worked to prevent the need for foster care by helping "at risk" families find housing and employment. They also publicized the condi-

tions and treatment of children at Junior Village and put significant pressure on the city to close the institution. Eventually, theirs and other efforts were successful. In 1973, Junior Village closed its doors for good.

25. The group included Paul and Ellen Peachey, Don and Sally White, Delton and Marian Franz, Bob and Esther Wert, Verle and Vivian Headings, Leroy and Jane Walters, Eva Beidler, and others on occasion.

26. In the Church of the Saviour, members would "sound a call" on a Sunday morning, describing a concern they believed God had placed in them. If at least one other person felt called to the same vision, they formed a mission group to begin fleshing out the call and bringing it to be. Even though not everyone in my parents' supper group was part of the Church of the Saviour, Vivian's call followed a similar model.

When I talk to Vivian, she plays down her role in the meeting my dad describes, emphasizing the *group* process. She tells the facts of the story a bit differently—as often happens with stories that are more than thirty years old—but she does agree that it was she who "piped up with fear and trembling," calling a group together to explore possibilities.

27. Margaret Wenger, Betty Louise Hershey, Dan Hess, Del Glick, and George Richards, who taught half-time

28. Name has been changed for reasons of confidentiality.

29. See Chapter 2.

30. See Chapter 6.

31. As of this publication, FLOC has downsized considerably, closing some of its programs and transferring a few others to different agencies. FLOC discontinued the Learning Center largely because of uncertain funding from the public school system. As it moves forward, FLOC is focusing its resources and staff energy on after-school programs and other educational initiatives.

32. Every year since 1990, activists have gathered in Fort Benning, Georgia, to call for the closing of the School of the Americas (which now bears a different name), a U.S.-funded military school whose graduates have been accused of perpetrating gruesome human rights violations, particularly in Latin America.

33. Dad tells some of Homestead's history later in this chapter. When the Rolling Ridge community began talking seriously about moving to the land, they had to decide what to communicate to the Jones family, who had been living on the land for years. It was a difficult discussion, but ultimately, the group decided to ask the Jones family to leave. In the years since, Homestead has undergone a facelift, mostly since Keith moved in, in 1993—complete with the addition of electricity, running water, lovely wooden beams, and a corn-burning stove. It is a lovely place.

34. Verle and Vivian Headings, Bob and Jackie Sabath, Trish Stefanik, and George Faix.

35. My parents had known Verle and Vivian for several years by now, particularly from the Mennonite group which met on Sunday evenings, and the

Learning Center support group. The Headings were very committed to the idea of intentional community. Even as the group of people who eventually founded Rolling Ridge and then supported it over the years has shifted and changed, Verle and Vivian have remained involved as anchors and visionaries.

36. Early on, the group included (in addition to my parents and the Headings) Bob and Esther Wert, Pete and Florence Mills, Dabney and Alta Miller, and Paul and Ellen Peachey, who brought a strong interest in study and retreat. Paul Peachey has also told some of the Rolling Ridge story in his own memoir, *A Usable Past? A Story of Living and Thinking Vocationally at the Margins* (Telford, Pa.: DreamSeeker Books/Cascadia, 2008).

37. The Niles soon created the Rolling Ridge Foundation. ("Yes," my dad acknowledged, "it was the Niles who came up with the name 'Rolling Ridge.' Our group later struggled and struggled to name our retreat project and eventually asked the foundation for permission to use their name, calling it the Rolling Ridge Study Retreat Community. The name really works. It's got a nice sound to it and kind of rolls, just like the landscape.") The number of acres belonging to the foundation has shifted and changed over the years, and now totals 1,400.

38. Tremba learned about the group because he attended Church of the Saviour, along with the Headings and the Millers.

39. Together they bought a tract of land that had one large house and a second, smaller house. At about the same time, Bob and Esther Wert were returning from two years in Kansas. They were interested in living in community with other families but did not share our interest in the study-retreat project. Their family joined the other two in the Shepherdstown community for only three years, sharing a house with the Headings, and then moved to Goshen, Indiana.

40. Also known as Hunter's Field

41. The Niles' Rolling Ridge Foundation wanted to lease the land to established entities, but in 1976, the little group of four families, to which my parents belonged, did not feel they were prepared to incorporate, so they made an arrangement with Church of the Saviour in Washington to sponsor them. In 1977, Church of the Saviour and the Rolling Ridge Foundation signed the original lease for 130 acres of land. The lease was written with language that assumed Church of the Saviour would transfer the land to a new entity within a few years, a transfer that did not actually happen until 1985 when the "core members" group was finally incorporated as a not-for-profit organization.

42. According to Dad, the Retreat House is actually too small to make a commercial program of retreats cost-effective. In order for a weekend retreat to pay for itself—for food, supplies, and a resource person to lead the retreat—it really requires more than twenty participants. The Retreat House has capacity for only fifteen.

43. Rolling Ridge later raised this amount to $3,600, to cover its costs.

44. *Faith Road to Rolling Ridge*, written by Tom Donlon in 1990, tells the

history of Rolling Ridge up to that point. The booklet was an important resource in finalizing this chapter as Dad was no longer living to check that facts and details were accurate. The booklet would be helpful to anyone interested in a more comprehensive account of the early history of Rolling Ridge. Copies are available through the Rolling Ridge Study Retreat Community, www.rollingridge.net.

45. Since Dad's death, several transitions have taken place in the Rolling Ridge residential community. Keith and Rachelle have moved to D.C. Billy and Lindsay McLaughlin, and Trish Stefanik have joined the community, moving into Pinestone and Homestead respectively. Scot and Linda DeGraf have also joined and are building the fifth and final community house.

46. The e-mail has been edited slightly from it's original length, but most of the content is the same.

47. The head covering, cape dress, and plain coat are all parts of traditional Mennonite dress that emphasize modesty, simplicity, and submission to God. My mother herself wore a head covering until she graduated from college. Today, plain dress is still practiced among conservative Mennonites, while it has all but disappeared from most Mennonite circles. The selection of ministers "by lot," another tradition that has fallen out of common practice, involved the nomination of men in the congregation when their church was in need of a minister. The nominees arrived on the day of ordination without knowing which of them would be chosen for the job. As the church filled with prayerful suspense, a bishop passed from man to man, opening the Bible each had picked up from a table at the front of the church to discover which man's Bible contained a slip of paper, designating him as the one chosen by God for ordination.

48. Even though Community House Church, the church my family attended, was nondenominational, it had strong ties to the Mennonite Church, as many in the group had grown up Mennonite. I also claimed that identity because of my strongly Mennonite family tree.

49. House Church is not void of belief statements. Every year, members commit and recommit to a Statement of Faith and Action, which reads, in part, "We affirm that God is the creator and sustainer of all life and in whose image humanity is created; that Jesus Christ through His life, death, and resurrection is the full revelation of God and the Lord of our lives; that God's Spirit is the guiding presence and comforter in our lives now; and that the Christian Church is a primary channel of God's love and presence in today's world." The ethos of the church, however, allows for considerable flexibility and question-asking within, around, and even overriding that statement. Still, while I praise the church's openness to different points of view, my mom calls the church a "rock" she can stand on. This Statement is part of her—and others'—rock.

50. Dan Charles, "Words at Nelson's Funeral—Nelson in House Church," July 2005.

51. And if House Church was a family, then by the time of his death, Dad was undoubtedly the patriarch. Some even asked—mostly in jest, I think—how the church would possibly go on without him, but it has indeed survived his loss and continues to meet today.

52. The melody to this Finnish hymn was composed in 1899 by Jean Sibelius. The words quoted here, which have been sung again and again by various artists and at assorted peace gatherings, were written in 1934 by Lloyd Stone, but the same melody is used in the traditional Christian hymn, "Be Still, My Soul," with words from a poem written in 1752 by Katharina von Schlegel and translated into English in 1855 by Jane Borthwick.

53. Dad took one year of classes at Millersville in Lancaster County, in between his freshman and junior years at Eastern Mennonite University in Harrisonburg, Virginia.

54. In 1976, as mentioned in note 22, Church of the Saviour divided into smaller sister churches because of its growing size. My parents attended Seekers Faith Community (one of these sister churches) somewhat regularly. Fred Taylor, who knew my parents from their work with the FLOC Learning Center, was the pastor at Seekers. David and Sharon Lloyd, who would move into my parents' house later that year, were also members.

55. My parents knew a number of them: Eva Beidler had been in voluntary service with them and had since married John Swarr; Arden and Maribeth Shank were good friends, in part because of Dad's work with Arden in the WSSY program; and my parents also knew Jim and Grace Dickerson, who had met in the city, moved to Arkansas, and recently returned. According to Dad's memory at the time of my interview with him, Terri and Tammy Colvin, Beth Burbank, and Sherri Murphy were also part of this original supper group.

56. Marlin and Barb Good's house, John Swarr and Eva Beidler's, and my parents'

57. Marlin was Dad's second cousin and served as the Learning Center's program director alongside Dad for a number of years. Our families are very close.

58. See Chapter 6.

59. This was, in part, a critique of the Church of the Saviour, which articulated its faith as having inward and outward dimensions.

60. Today, the church Jim and Grace started in the Shaw neighborhood of northwest Washington is known as New Community Church and is a part of the Church of the Saviour network.

61. Elders are the lay leaders in many Mennonite congregations, working closely with the paid pastor.

62. For Love of Children (FLOC) was founded in 1965 to serve troubled families and foster children. For more details on the organization and my dad's history with it, see Chapter 3.

63. The words were written by FLOC Board chair, Kate Cudlipp, June 2001.

64. All memories of the farewell party are from my mom, who was present for the occasion.

65. Fred Taylor retired as Executive Director of FLOC in December 2002.

66. In all this, Dad worked in collaboration with Kay Schultz and Missy Horning from a housing nonprofit called Manna.

67. The new organization was called the Anthony Bowen Landmark Building Trust.

68. The nonprofit they formed is now called the Thurgood Marshall Center Trust. A housing nonprofit called Manna was also involved in the project and actually paid my dad's paycheck, out of government funding they received for approved projects.

69. Respectively: executive director of FLOC, president of the Thurgood Marshall Center Trust, and chairman of the Shaw Heritage Trust

70. Prior to his work as a construction manager, Jair Lynch had been a U.S. Olympic silver medalist in gymnastics, a fact that I think Dad enjoyed repeating (not everyone gets to work closely with an Olympic medalist).

71. Thomasina Yearwood

72. As of this publication, FLOC has downsized considerably, closed the Learning Center, and moved its offices from the Thurgood Marshall Center to a smaller facility. Other nonprofit organizations have taken its place in the historic building.

73. As noted in Chapter 2, Dad was the primary visionary in founding the Washington Study-Service Year (WSSY) program of Eastern Mennonite College (EMC) in 1976. In the years since, EMC became EMU and, in 2002, WSSY became WCSC, the Washington Community Scholars' Center.

74. Kimberly Schmidt, "Cracking the Facility Nut," *Service Matters: An Alumni Newsletter of the WCSC,* Summer 2005.

75. At the time of my interview with Dad, the WCSC (formerly WSSY) program was still located in the original stucco house on South Dakota Avenue. As described in Chapter 2, the house had been a voluntary service house until Eastern Board decided to close the unit in 1975. The following year, the first group of WSSY students moved in. In 1979, EMC bought the house from Eastern Board for a very modest price, and the WSSY/WCSC program continued to use the building for nearly three decades in all.

76. May 2005

77. The new building, now called the Nelson Good House, was completed several months after Dad died, and students moved in on January 3, 2006.

78. Excerpt from "The Hardest Work You Will Ever Do," ©2005 Mary Cook. Used with permission of This I Believe, Inc. (www.thisibelieve.org).

THE AUTHOR

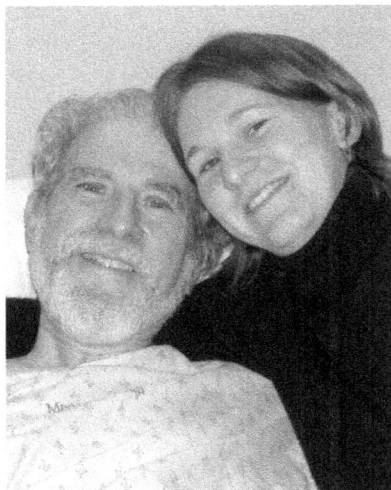

At twenty-four, Deborah Good was living in Philadelphia, Pennsylvania, when her life was hit suddenly with unexpected, terrible news. She was standing next to her dad, who lay in a stretcher outside the emergency room, when Doctor Noel filled them in: The CT-scans showed a mass on his left adrenal gland, spots on his lungs and liver.

It was, they would learn, a rare and aggressive form of cancer called adrenocortical carcinoma. In the tumultuous week that followed the diagnosis, Deborah moved back in with her parents, Betty and Nelson Good, in Washington, D.C. She joined with her mom in caring for her dad as best they knew how.

As Nelson approached death, Deborah spent hours sitting with her dad as he reflected back on the interlocking pieces of his unconventional job life. Admittedly, Nelson was neither a saint nor a celebrity and, by many measures, was a rather ordinary guy, yet he lived with a humble integrity and a commitment to others that touched many people. During his four decades in the city, he became committed to building small communities and organizations—a radical act in a world increasingly dominated by the belief that *bigger* was better.

From his spot on a padded green recliner, Nelson told the stories, one at a time, of seven projects, communities, and orga-

nizations he had cared deeply about: a neighborhood community center, an experiential education program for college students, an alternative day school for foster children, a retreat
center, a house church, a historic building restoration, and a
unique house renovation.

He moistened his mouth with water as he spoke, and Deborah listened, took notes, and tape-recorded their conversations. Later, she would add her own reflections in between his.
The resulting memoir is a unique intertwining of a father's history-telling with a daughter's personal journey of remembrance, loss, and grief.

www.ingramcontent.com/pod-product-compliance
Lightning Source LLC
Chambersburg PA
CBHW030010290326
41934CB00005B/283